EMS
Street
Strategies

EMS
Street
Strategies
Effective Patient Interaction

SECOND EDITION

Stephen Michael Soreff, M.D.
President, Education Initiatives, Worcester, MA
Lecturer, UMassMemorial Emergency Medical Services, Worcester, MA
Faculty, Boston University-Metropolitan College, Boston, MA
Mount Wachusett Community College, Leominster, MA
Fisher College, Boston, MA
Director of Quality Improvement, HMA Behavioral Health, Worcester, MA

Robert T. Cadigan, Ph.D.
Associate Professor
Criminal Justice and Sociology
Metropolitan College, Boston University

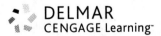

DELMAR
CENGAGE Learning

Australia • Brazil • Japan • Korea • Mexico • Singapore • Spain • United Kingdom • United States

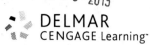

DELMAR
CENGAGE Learning™

**EMS Street Strategies: Effective
Patient Interaction,
Second Edition**
Stephen Michael Soreff
and Robert T. Cadigan

Health Care Publishing Director:
William Brottmiller

Executive Editor: Cathy L. Esperti

Acquisitions Editor: Maureen
Rosener

Developmental Editor:
Darcy M. Scelsi

Editorial Assistant:
Matthew Thouin

Executive Marketing Manager:
Dawn F. Gerrain

Channel Manager: Gretta Oliver

Production Editor: James Zayicek

For product information and
technology assistance, contact us at **Cengage Learning
Customer & Sales Support, 1-800-354-9706**

For permission to use material from this text or product,
submit all requests online at **www.cengage.com/
permissions** Further permissions questions can be emailed
to **permissionrequest@cengage.com**

Library of Congress Control Number: 2002035198

ISBN-13: 978-0-7668-2013-5

ISBN-10: 0-7668-2013-0

Delmar
Executive Woods
5 Maxwell Drive
Clifton Park, NY 12065
USA

Cengage Learning is a leading provider of customized learning
solutions with office locations around the globe, including
Singapore, the United Kingdom, Australia, Mexico, Brazil, and
Japan. Locate your local office at
international.cengage.com/region

Cengage Learning products are represented in Canada by
Nelson Education, Ltd.

To learn more about Delmar, visit **www.cengage.com/delmar**

Purchase any of our products at your local bookstore or at our
preferred online store **www.ichapters.com**

Notice to the Reader
Publisher does not warrant or guarantee any of the products described herein or perform any independent analysis in connection
with any of the product information contained herein. Publisher does not assume, and expressly disclaims, any obligation to obtain
and include information other than that provided to it by the manufacturer. The reader is expressly warned to consider and adopt
all safety precautions that might be indicated by the activities described herein and to avoid all potential hazards. By following the
instructions contained herein, the reader willingly assumes all risks in connection with such instructions. The publisher makes no representations or warranties of any kind, including but not limited to, the warranties of fitness for particular purpose or merchantability,
nor are any such representations implied with respect to the material set forth herein, and the publisher takes no responsibility with
respect to such material. The publisher shall not be liable for any special, consequential, or exemplary damages resulting, in whole or

Printed in the United States of America
5 6 7 8 9   16 15 14 13 12

FD170

*To my daughters, Sasha and Matana, and to my sons, Ben and Barak,
to my partner, Peggy, to my sister, Linda, and to the adventurous
spirit of where we have not gone before.*
SMS

To my wife, Doris, our sons, Philip and Patrick, and our daughter, Laurie.
RTC

*And to the professional, dedicated, and compassionate men and women of
Emergency Medical Services.*

CONTENTS

FOREWORD... ix

PREFACE... xi

ACKNOWLEDGMENTS.. xiii

ABOUT THE AUTHORS....................................... xiv

CHAPTER 1   Introduction 1

CHAPTER 2   Cardiac Emergency: The Heart of the Matter......... 11

CHAPTER 3   The Elderly: Handle with Care.................... 23

CHAPTER 4   AIDS: A Fatal Virus............................. 41

CHAPTER 5   Trauma: More Than Physical Injury................ 51

CHAPTER 6   Rape: Hidden Injuries 63

CHAPTER 7   The Brutalized Child: A Family in Despair 75

CHAPTER 8   The Potentially Violent Patient: Anxiety, Ambivalence, and Aggression 89

CHAPTER 9   Depression and Suicide: A Semester in Hell......... 105

CHAPTER 10   Alcohol Abuse: Broken Bottles, Broken Dreams...... 117

CHAPTER 11   The Unwanted: Deinstitutionalization, Detoxification, and Dereliction of Duty 133

CHAPTER 12   Provocative Patients: The Sexy, the Suit Conscious, and the Somatizing 143

CHAPTER 13   Responding to All People: EMS in the Era of Diversity 163

CHAPTER 14   Death in the Ambulance: Grief and Guilt........... 177

CHAPTER 15   Multiple Casualty Incident: The Demands, Destruction, and Disorientation................. 189

CHAPTER 16   Street and System Stresses: Recognition Is the Key ... 199

CHAPTER 17 EMS Wellness: Things You Can Do to Help Yourself
Handle Stress Better 215

ANSWERS TO REVIEW QUESTIONS 231

GLOSSARY 237

INDEX 243

FOREWORD

One of the cardinal rules taught in each emergency medical training program from First Responder through Paramedic is, Save the Rescuer First. This message has seen us through Hazardous Materials scenarios, Bloodborne Pathogens exposures, an AIDS/HIV education crisis, and failure to recognize the cumulative effects of critical incident stress. Still we have a cadre of almost 1 million committed career and volunteer EMS professionals who continue to provide this nation with a prehospital emergency response system that is barely matched in most industrialized nations.

Nearly 20 years ago, while doing research for my graduate degree, I discovered that there was a 50 percent attrition rate over a 3-year period among advanced life support providers in the New York county where I was doing my research. I went on to discover that the entire state of New York had a similar rate and it ran the gamut from first responders, emergency medical technicians, advanced EMTs to paramedics. More research led me to believe that this attrition rate was a problem across the nation, not easily distinguished by career, volunteer, or mixed service; urban, suburban, or rural setting; or any other work load-based identifier I was able to discern. Sadly, after almost an entire career as a prehospital provider, having seen numerous attempts at retention programs, both local and statewide, these attrition rates remain ominously constant today.

That high attrition rate is why this book is so critically important. Its premise is to provide skills, options, awareness, and opportunities that will enhance the sustainability of the emergency medical services workforce. With a daunting new array of risks confronting us, from antibiotic-resistant tuberculosis to the now very real threat of exposure to biological or chemical weapons of mass effect, prehospital care providers no longer only witness the struggle between life and death, they have become at-risk participants. In fact, in too many cases they may even have become the primary targets of terrorists' secondary devices.

EMS providers stand at the crossroads of two career paths: public safety and public health. They bring the most special attributes of both to their patients: the courage and daring of the public safety sector and the caring and compassion of the public health community. Within these pages lies the information necessary to maintain that commitment to community, homeland, and nation. In the post-September 11, 2001 world, there is a need to upgrade our skills, enhance our knowledge base, expand our practice capabilities, and, most important, increase the likelihood of returning safely to our families after responding to each call for help. Former Governor Tom Ridge, now the nation's Director of Homeland Security, has called America's law enforcement, firefighters, and emergency medical personnel "the front-line soldiers in the event of a terrorist attack." With the next federal budget reflecting a 1,000 percent increase in the funds available to states and localities for enhancing their response capabilities, we must remember that our most important assets are the providers themselves.

Please use this revised and updated text as a tool for retaining and preserving the practiced provider and for extending the service life of new providers. Medical judgment, perhaps the most important skill of a prehospital provider, cannot be taught in a classroom; it must be learned by experience. Even if there were an endless line of candidates waiting to become EMS providers, which we know does not exist, failure to maintain our experienced providers condemns the next generation to learn not from our mistakes, but rather from making their own—a senseless, time-consuming, and patient-unfriendly practice, that works against our wish to be perceived as professionals and one that likely will contribute to maintaining the disturbingly high rate of attrition among us. Use these pages as a primer of potential pitfalls that can be avoided by knowledge and awareness of them. Share this information with your officers, peers, and, most importantly, your "newbies" so they may become your service's "worker bees" in the shortest amount of time possible. The days of sending the probie to the rig to retrieve a piece of equipment, when he or she is the least likely to know where it is, have passed, along with the Cadillac ambulance and the Thomas half-ring splint. Our determination to be perceived by other members of the health-care community as professionals requires this sharing.

The public has increasing expectations from their prehospital providers. We must find those with the intelligence, desire, and compassion to replenish our depleted ranks. Ralph Waldo Emerson said: "What lies behind us and what lies before us are tiny matters compared to what lies within us." I take these sage words of wisdom to each ambulance call, squad meeting, and training session. Use each chapter of this text as a lesson in survival for both you and your agency membership. In the immortal words of the roll call sergeant from Hill Street Blues: "Let's be careful out there."

Martin H. Singer, M.P.S.
Coordinator Hospital Bioterrorism Preparedness
Pennsylvannia Department of Health

PREFACE

In the rubble of the World Trade Center, in the flood waters of North Carolina, in the smoke of Columbine, in the broken glass of Oklahoma City, in the earthquake collapse of San Francisco's Marina District, in the frozen fields of the Northeast ice storm, and in the aftermath of hurricane Andrew a picture of the heroic, dedicated, and caring EMS provider stands. The images of the EMS provider that emerge best captures how the world has changed for them and for us since the first edition of *EMS Street Strategies* in 1992. One of the greatest symbols of that transformation remains the National EMS Memorial established in 1992 in Roanoke, Virginia, and dedicated to those EMS providers who have died in the line of duty.

In the last 10 years the world and the health-care world have both dramatically changed and have remained the same. The health-care industry has seen major changes: improved medical and surgical treatments and techniques, new generations of medications, the rise of managed care; the increase in private and public emergency response programs, the growth of the elderly population, the greatly expanded diversity of America, the substantial number of people without health insurance coverage, the newer technologies, the development of the Internet, the number of persons with HIV/AIDS, and the heightened threats to our personal and national safety and security. At the same time, people in emergencies face death, disfigurement, destruction, and dangers with the same sense of urgency, fear of death, disability and disfigurement, terror, apprehension and uncertainty as they have in the past. Still EMS providers confront daily their own blood, tears, and pain as they always have.

The mission of the book remains to offer the EMS provider an understanding of the person and the personality in the midst of the crisis and to furnish the responders with a solid step-by-step method to intervene effectively and efficiently. Each chapter commences with a scenario depicting real situations. We focus on the origins of behavior and offer a proven intervention sequence of "Observe," "Interaction," "Ask," "Act," "Attend," and "Document." We have incorporated the changes in a number of ways. We have included chapters on the elderly, population diversity, and wellness. We have added exercises and answers to the review questions. We have expanded the references with Internet information, movies, books, and articles.

However, the interaction between EMS providers and patients stands as the heart of the intervention and enhancing that connection remains the core value of *EMS Street Strategies*. The tradition of people helping people based on their skills, professionalism, and dedication is the cornerstone of this book. We provide the provider with key knowledge and techniques to advance and improve that interaction and that care. In the end, this book helps EMS providers pay more and better attention to the patient and the patient's family and significantly more attention to themselves.

ACKNOWLEDGMENTS

We could not have achieved the quality of this volume without the support, and perseverence of many people. First, and foremost our developmental editor, Darcy Scelsi. Her wisdom, judgment and attention to detail has guided us in this undertaking. We are indebted to the very helpful insights provided by the reviewers of the second edition. We especially are grateful to Richard Beebe and Deborah Funk for their book *Fundamentals of Emergency Care,* which demonstrated the way the psychosocial dimensions have been incorporated into the mainstream of EMS work and texts.

A number of others have been extremely helpful in the development of this edition. Marc Restuccia, M.D., FACEP, Medical Director, UMassMemorial EMS/Lifeflight provided key references. Richard Wetherbee, R.N., EMT-P, EMS supervisor, UMassMemorial furnished some very nifty and useful Internet sites. Patricia Ball, R.N., offered some super movie ideas. Jacqueline Belrose, Dean of Lifelong Learning and Workforce Development, Mount Wachusett Community College supplied some key legal Internet sites.

ABOUT THE AUTHORS

Stephen Soreff, M.D., is a nationally known health-care lecturer, author, and experiential learning innovator. He has lectured throughout the United States on a wide variety of psychiatric topics, including aggression, suicide, stress management, and quality improvement.

Dr. Soreff is the psychiatric editor in chief of the psychiatric section of the e-medicine online *Medicine, Surgical, Obstetrical and Psychiatric* e-text book. As well as a lecturer at UMass Memorial Emergency Medical Service, he is on the faculty of many New England colleges and universities, including Metropolitan College, Boston University, Mount Wachusett Community College, and Fisher College. He has been a guest lecturer in a Harvard University Medical School program. He is on the faculty of the W.I.S.E. program—Worcester's Institute for Senior Education—and often lectures at Massachusetts School of Professional Psychology.

In 1994, Dr. Soreff founded Education Initiatives with its mission to provide in-house, in-services to nursing facilities. He received the Walter E. Barton, M.D. Award from the American College of Mental Health Administration for his research on quality improvement. He has authored numerous books and articles on mental illness, emergency medical services, documentation, and communication. Dr. Soreff also produces and hosts two radio programs providing consumers with the most up-to-date medical information.

Robert T. Cadigan, Ph.D., is associate professor of Criminal Justice and Sociology, Metropolitan College, Boston University. He was formerly director of training in the Massachusetts Office of Emergency Medical Services. Dr. Cadigan is coauthor of two studies of violence against Emergency Medical Services providers and coauthor of a management workbook for volunteer ambulance service managers.

CHAPTER 1

Introduction

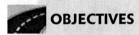 **OBJECTIVES**

Upon completion of this chapter, you should be able to:

- Discuss the importance of communication and interpersonal skills as they relate to improving patient care.
- Demonstrate an understanding of the patient's world and the patient's actions in a given scenario.
- Demonstrate an understanding of the emergency medical services (EMS) provider's response within a given scenario and discuss the importance of maintaining unbiased care.

THE CHALLENGE

As EMS enters the 21st century, we face challenges that were unheard of, or ignored, a decade ago. The most dramatic, though not necessarily the most difficult, challenge is coming to grips with the threat of domestic terrorism. The most pervasive is working within a health system in crisis. Ambulance services are under increasing financial pressure as reimbursement rates have not kept pace with costs, and government support for EMS systems is declining. Hospitals are closing, emergency departments are turning away ambulances, and patients are either not being admitted or are being discharged sooner—and probably sicker—than at any other time in recent history. Other more subtle changes are those in patient populations. Deinstitutionalization of formerly hospitalized psychiatric patients, mainstreaming of persons with disabilities, the increasing diversity of the population, and the increasing numbers of elderly are creating new challenges. These patients may not only challenge our technical skills but also challenge us to reach out to persons who are different from us.

While it may seem obvious that we need to pay more attention to patients as persons, technical skill training takes increasing time. There seems to be less time to focus on basic patient care both in training and in practice. Training in intravenous therapy and automatic defibrillation are standard or widely adopted optional skills for many basic EMS providers. As valuable as these therapies may be in well-designed systems of care, it is important to balance technical sophistication with interpersonal skills to handle the challenge of change.[1] The goal of this book is to improve your understanding of patients and your interpersonal skills as a caregiver.

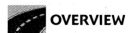 ## OVERVIEW

We have identified 16 challenging patient care situations, ranging from working with the unstable chest pain patient to dealing with death and disaster. For each of these, we present a scenario, "The Patient and the Situation," and describe

- The patient's world
- The behavior of the patient
- The emotions and thoughts behind the behavior
- Family/bystander responses
- Provider responses
- Intervention strategies
- Considerations for EMS providers

In some chapters we provide additional background on the causes of the behavior involved. For example, to understand why an alcoholic drinks, you must understand **alcoholism** as a disease; to understand the relationship between **depression** and suicide, it is necessary to understand the dynamics of depression. When we discuss chronic disease or child abuse, we consider family dynamics and their effect on the emergency situation.

 ## THE PATIENT AND THE SITUATION

Each chapter, or major section, begins with a **vignette** describing a fictional emergency. In these stories, you meet patients and their families. The vignette provides a springboard for discussion of the behavior of the patient and the emotions and thoughts behind that behavior. We do not mean to stereotype patients but rather to raise your awareness of the hidden dynamics of emergency intervention. We agree with psychiatrist Robert Coles when he says that we can learn much from stories and our reactions to them.[2] This is the way that most people throughout history have learned: stories encourage us to confront and consider our values, attitudes, and behavior as well as giving us insights into the values, attitudes, and behavior of others.

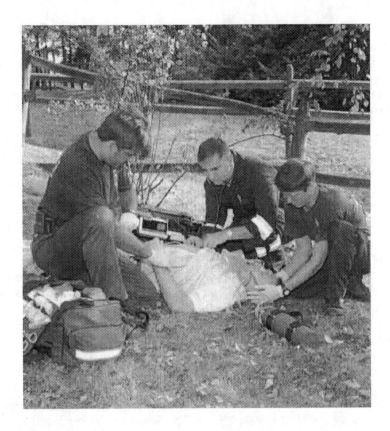

Our fictional heroes and heroines are not perfect. We hope we have been honest in presenting real-life attitudes and actions. **Cynicism, anxiety** over working with persons with communicable diseases, and frustration in working with homeless persons are real issues. In the case presentation or discussion, we may suggest ways in which care could have been improved. To keep our focus on interaction, we have generally limited descriptions of assessment and treatment procedures. The standard texts define the core knowledge you must have in these cases. We include standard references at various points in our chapters. Of course, you must follow the standards of care established in your state or region for your level of certification.

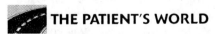 **THE PATIENT'S WORLD**

To treat a patient effectively, you must enter his or her world. Many patients are experiencing levels of pain and anxiety that most EMS providers have never experienced. Some anxiety is directly related to the patient's chief complaint; some is related to being dependent on others. Communicating with a patient in pain can be difficult. It can be especially difficult when the patient is from a different ethnic or economic background or is significantly older or younger than you. You cannot expect the patient to understand your world, but as part of your professional orientation, you must attempt to appreciate the patient's world. In "The Patient's World" section, we suggest some of the conditions surrounding the patient that can affect your ability to relate, assess, and treat. A violence-prone patient (Chapter 8), an alcoholic patient (Chapter 10), or an abused child (Chapter 7) and his or her family members live in a world in which family relationships and relationships with neighbors may be organized very differently than in a functional family. A victim of sudden illness (Chapter 2) or injury (Chapters 5 and 6) lives in a very different world than that of a person suffering from chronic disease (Chapter 4).

 ## THE BEHAVIOR OF THE PATIENT

For many patients, the crisis that results in an emergency call is unprecedented. A patient with a condition as common as a sprained ankle can demonstrate out-of-control behavior that seems disproportionate to the pain or to the severity of the injury. Because a patient appears to be responding personally to you, you may not appreciate how that behavior is determined more by the situation than by anything you have done. We look at common behavioral patterns often seen in a particular type of emergency. A victim of rape (Chapter 6) may alternate between accepting and rejecting offered help; the son or the spouse of a person who has died in the ambulance may react violently to the news of the death (Chapter 14). These all represent normal responses to abnormal situations. In other situations, abnormal responses may be the reason for the emergency call: an abusing parent has seriously injured a child (Chapter 7); a depressed college student has overdosed on alcohol and medication (Chapter 9); an alcoholic patient causes problems in a residential neighborhood (Chapter 10).

 ## THE EMOTIONS AND THOUGHTS BEHIND THE BEHAVIOR

Emotions and thoughts generally precede and explain observed behavior. Many behaviors that a dying patient exhibits are related to which emotional stage of coming to grips with death the patient is in (Chapter 4). Many other behaviors that appear baffling, such a denial of pain or illness, may be typical or habitual responses related to the patient's psychologic state or persistent traits. The lawsuit-conscious patient or the **sexually provocative** patient who appears to be responding to the EMS provider may be acting on emotions and thoughts developed in response to a wide variety of other situations (Chapter 12). The potentially violent patient (Chapter 8) who poses a direct physical threat may be drawing cues from thoughts and emotions unrelated to what you are doing.

By understanding the connections between emotions/thoughts and behavior, you will feel more comfortable and confident in deescalating the potentially dangerous situation.

 ## FAMILY/BYSTANDER RESPONSES

Families and bystanders often influence emergency care. Families, especially, have their own concerns and attitudes that will affect you and the patient. When treating a patient experiencing chest pain in his home (Chapter 2), you may find yourself surrounded by concerned but confused family members who do not understand what you are doing. In many cases, families will feel somehow responsible for the situation because they have either ignored or minimized the patient's medical complaints (Chapter 3). Bystanders can either be allies or create problems. Looking at the scene from the bystander's perspective can sometimes help you to communicate in the patient's best interest (Chapter 10).

 ## PROVIDER RESPONSES

As well as understanding patient responses to emergencies, you must be sensitive to your own responses to patients in distress. This self-awareness is the beginning of deeper wisdom and mastery over challenging situations. We discuss specific ways in which working with or working through your reactions will improve the care you provide.

It is important to approach the scene without **preconceptions**. On one hand, if you stereotype a neighborhood, family, or patient based on past experiences or hearsay, you are denying that patient the professional approach that he or she deserves. Chapter 13, Responding to All People, deals with stereotypes and prejudice. Yet, on the other hand, by your recognizing prior actions in that area or with that household, you are actually using that information to promote your own safety. If you prejudge a case as a psychiatric emergency, a diabetic emergency, or "only" a routine transfer, you can limit your effectiveness and endanger a patient. While we feel that most EMS providers will benefit from the information that dispatchers gather and pass on, it is important to rely on your own senses and intuitions in approaching, entering, and managing a scene.

 ## INTERVENTION STRATEGIES

In "Intervention Strategies" we suggest techniques that will help you to approach each assessment and treatment with fresh eyes. Our concern is with observation and interaction techniques, not patient care skills such as splinting, spineboarding, or starting a intravenous (IV) line. However, your comfort with the assessment process and your technical proficiency foster patient confidence that is necessary for effective interaction. Being professional begins with hands-on skills and includes the ability to perform competently regardless of personal feelings about the patient or the situation. The intervention section suggests specific courses of action to take in the emergency care situation described in the chapter.

We identify six common components in each intervention:

- Observe
- Interact
- Ask
- Act
- Attend
- Document

Box 1–1 briefly summarizes each of these components.

Observe

Observing involves sizing up the scene and, where relevant, determining likely mechanisms of injury while approaching the patient. Approaching any scene involves threats to personal safety. Certain situations represent particularly dangerous threats such as an accident on a busy thoroughfare or working with an intoxicated patient. In other cases, such as approaching a depressed patient (Chapter 9) or abused child (Chapter 7), special features of the environment are important for your patient assessment and care.

Interact

Interacting relates to your general approach to the patient or patient's family. Your general appearance and tone in approaching a possible heart attack victim

---

BOX 1–1

COMPONENTS OF EMERGENCY CARE

Observe	Size up the scene and approach safely.
Interact	Establish rapport with the patient and significant others.
Ask	Determine the patient's chief complaint, current status, and significant medical history.
Act	Provide emergency care.
Attend	Listen effectively to what the patient has to say.
Document	Describe the care provided.

(Chapter 2) or a person with acquired immunodeficiency syndrome (AIDS) (Chapter 4) can affect patient cooperation and compliance. Your appearance and tone in approaching a sexually provocative patient or a patient who seems intent on suing someone (Chapter 12) can save you embarrassment or legal difficulty, as well as assure an effective treatment.

Ask

Asking includes investigating the patient's current complaint and medical history. There are common tricks of the trade that will help you in all patient encounters. The OPQRST technique for assessing pain in described in Chapter 2; the SAMPLE technique of history taking is described in Chapter 3. The questions you ask and the order in which you ask them will affect the quality of the information you receive. We recommend some common strategies (Chapter 2) for interviewing patients concerning the history of their present illness and pain. However, there are other tricks of the trade that are important in special situations, such as your approach to a child (Chapter 7) or geriatric patient (Chapter 3).

Act

Acting refers to the physical interventions you must perform. Physical care is at the heart of your service to the patient, whether a homeless person (Chapter 11) or a trauma patient (Chapter 15).

Attend

Attending is listening—really listening—to what the patient has to say. This skill is neglected but is one that is important for effective care in every patient encounter. It is especially difficult, however, when the patient may arouse negative feelings in you. It means being with the patient through the entire intervention. In Chapter 4 we discuss some characteristics of effective listening.

Document

Your job is not finished until the paperwork is done. There are specifics that must be recorded on every run. These include times, patient-identifying information, vital signs, assessment findings, spinal precautions, oxygen (if used), and other care rendered. It may also be important to note the contributions of, or complications caused by, others at the scene. In addition, some challenging care situations present special demands. The results of an assessment on a **somatizing** patient (Chapter 12), or **hypochondriac,** must be thoroughly documented even though the results of the assessment are negative. In caring for a suicidal patient (Chapter 9), you must gather information about the patient's potential danger to self and others and document such information.

One of the myths that has grown up in EMS is that no one reads the patient care report. This myth is not true. The patient care report is a major legal as well as medical document. Remember, if it is not documented, it did not happen!

CONSIDERATIONS FOR EMS PROVIDERS

Throughout, a professional approach to caring for a patient is crucial. While there are many different ways of defining professionalism, on scene, it will include, as John Becknell suggests:

- Valuing yourself and what you do
- Doing the best for those you help[3]

At the scene, you are called on to do the best for both the patient and the family. After the run, you must do the best for yourself. This effort includes honest review of your behavior, thoughts, and emotions. This exercise is important both to release **post-traumatic stress** and to open the way for future growth. A wise man once said, "There is a great deal of difference between having twenty years of experience and having one year of experience twenty times." In each chapter we conclude with some practical suggestions for EMS providers. We conclude the book (Chapters 17 and 18) with a discussion of stress and wellness for EMS providers.

CONCLUSION

Effective patient care depends on being able to think forward and backward from the immediate situation: to recognize the patient as an individual with a history that you must respect and a future that you will influence. Appreciating both the common features of patients and their individuality will keep your assessments sharp and your interest strong.

REVIEW QUESTIONS

1. How are thoughts, emotions, and behavior interrelated?
2. What are some conditions that may make it difficult for an EMS provider to communicate successfully with a patient?
3. List and define the six components common to every intervention.

EXERCISES

1. Interview a seasoned EMS provider about a memorable patient encounter. What was it that made the encounter stick in this EMS provider's mind? Ask about the behavior of the patient, the family, bystanders. Is the behavior of anyone involved what made this experience memorable? How did the EMS provider feel after this encounter?

2. After you have finished a shift with your local EMS unit, sit and write down the behaviors you observed in the patients, families, and bystanders you attended to that day. How did these behaviors impact patient care? Did they made the situation better or worse? Why?

3. Write down your feelings and expectations about the field of EMS. Do you have any preconceived notions about the job, your service area, your coworkers? Why do you feel this way? How do you think your feelings and expectations will impact your interactions with patients and coworkers?

4. What are some of the effects that the practice of emergency medical service can have on providers?

A NOTE ON REFERENCES

We have used references from EMS journals and publications in addition to other sources. We hope to encourage you to look into these journals and to use them as valuable tools for your professional growth in the future. In addition, there are general bibliographic citations from medical, psychiatric, and other scientific journals.

REFERENCES

1. Halley, A. A., Kopp, J., & Austin, J. (1998). *Delivering human services* (4th ed., pp. 545–562). New York: Longmans.

2. Coles, R. (1989). *The call of stories.* Boston: Houghton Mifflin.

3. Becknell, J. (1987). Discovering professionalism in EMS. *Journal of Emergency Medical Services, 12* (12) 30–32.

FURTHER INFORMATION

Internet Resources

Emergency Medical Technician Paramedic National Standard Curriculum: www.nhtsa.dot.gov/people/injury/ems/EMT-P/index.html

Great EMS Web site: www.defrance.org

Great health information entry point: www.WebMD.com

Dr. C. Everett Koop's site: www.drkoop.com

Medical textbook online: www.emedicine.com

Merck Manual: www.merck.com

National Association of Emergency Medical Physicians:
www.naemsp.org

National Institutes of Health: www.nih.gov/health

National EMS Memorial Web site: www.nemsms.org

Prehospital Emergency Care, online journal: www.peconline.org

Media Resources

Movies
Bringing Out the Dead

Mother, Jugs and Speed

Books
Beebe, R., & Funk, D. (2001). *Fundamentals of emergency care.* Clifton Park, NY: Delmar Learning.

Harwood, A., & Wolfson, A. B. (2001). *The clinical practice of emergency medicine,* 3d ed. Baltimore: Lippincott Williams and Wilkins.

Whittle, J. (2001). *911 Responding for life, case studies in emergency care.* Clifton Park, NY: Delmar Learning.

Cardiac Emergency
The Heart of the Matter

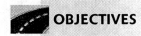 **OBJECTIVES**

Upon completion of this chapter, you should be able to:

- Understand the significance of coronary heart disease in the population and in your work.
- Describe the psychological significance of denial and minimization for a person who may be experiencing a heart attack.
- Understand how family anxiety and guilt may affect bystander response to EMS care.
- Show how you can adapt your intervention to the specific needs of the patient who may be experiencing a heart attack.
- Identify and learn to counteract EMS provider behaviors that can limit your effectiveness.

THE CHALLENGE

Approximately 7 million Americans have **coronary heart disease (CHD)**. Approximately 5 hundred thousand will die this year from heart attacks caused by CHD.[1] The basic cause of an **acute myocardial infarction** is a sudden reduction in or total occlusion of the blood supply to the heart muscle. A major interruption in the heart's blood supply can result in muscle damage, arrhythmias, and **congestive heart failure** (CHF).

There are three distinct psychosocial challenges in the emergency care of a person with a possible heart attack:

1. Responding to the patient's behavior. The patient may deny or minimize the severity of the symptoms or may be overwhelmed by anxiety over those symptoms.

11

2. Responding to the patient's family. Family reactions, including guilt and self-doubt, can influence their involvement.

3. Dealing with EMS stress. You must stay focused despite the reactions of patient and family.

Because chest pain is a relatively common chief complaint, you must be familiar with cardiac assessment and treatment procedures. However, the cardiac patient challenges our interpersonal skills as well as technical care skills.[2]

 THE PATIENT AND THE SITUATION

Forty-year-old Ken Jefferson feels a slight discomfort in his chest. He had a mild back pain a couple of days ago, but he has never felt a pain like this before. It's indigestion, he tells himself, and he attempts to concentrate on the newspaper.

He is sitting at the dining room table in his modestly furnished suburban home. He tries to read the sports page, but he cannot concentrate. He is still upset by his latest argument with his 16-year-old daughter, Brenda. Ken finds her latest boyfriend lazy and rude. He was upset to find out that Brenda had a date on a school night. However, when Ken found out that her book report on *Silas Marner* was not done, he curtailed her evening plans. In the middle of supper she fled to her room in a flurry of tears. She slammed the door decisively behind her. Ken's wife, Janet, ignored the interruption; their 12-year-old son Tony took the opportunity to show that he wanted to do well in school. He asked his father to help him with his upcoming science project. Ken begged off, saying of course he would, but not tonight, because of the office work he had to do.

Ken pushed aside the last of a scotch and water. As Janet went to clear the dishes from the table, she noted that Ken looked distant. She touched his arm. His skin seemed moist. She asked, "All right, dear?" He didn't hear her at first, as he had already—mentally—gone back to the shop. Since his promotion to foreman, he felt caught in the middle between his old friends and his new col-

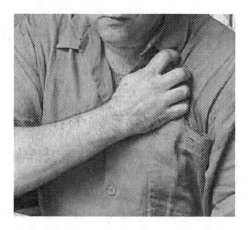

leagues in management. His family found him unapproachable. Ken looked at his watch. He has become highly time oriented. It was 6:37 P.M. He starts to work on next month's shop schedule.

By 6:45 P.M., he cannot ignore the pain. He thinks, briefly, of his father who died of a heart attack when Ken was 18, but he quickly dismisses such foolishness. He is becoming short of breath. He cannot concentrate on what he is trying to do. He wants to call for help, but he thinks, "What if it's just indigestion or muscle strain, or something trivial? Maybe my worrying about it is making me think it is worse than it really is. What will the doctor say? I didn't take her advice on dieting or smoking. Dr. Bennet is home with her family at supper. I can't call now."

Janet returns and sees his distress. She asks, "Are you OK?" He hesitates to answer, fearing another lecture about smoking too much. He gets up slowly and says, "I've got to lie down." Ken hunches forward and clutches at his chest as he moves. Janet decides whatever is wrong, he needs help. She calls Dr. Bennet's office. Her answering service says that they will try to contact the doctor, but in the meantime, Janet should get an ambulance. She calls 911 and reports that her husband is weak, short of breath, and clutching his chest when he moves.

The dispatcher promptly dispatches advanced life support and suggests that she help her husband into a semireclining position and assures her that help is on the way.

Brenda and Tony sense something is happening downstairs. When Brenda comes into the living room she wonders if her behavior has anything to do with her father's state. Tony is frightened when he sees his father breathing so strangely. He feels helpless.

Brenda tries to comfort her father, but the pain is becoming unbearable. He brushes her aside. She takes this rejection personally. Janet calls the doctor's answering service to find out why someone hasn't called back yet. It has only been 3 minutes since she made the first call, but it seems like an eternity.

EMS providers Linda Kingsford and Donald Thornton had just finished dinner when they received the call. Don fears he is a prime candidate for heart trouble down the line; even at age 35, his muscle is turning to fat and his doctor is warning him about borderline hypertension.

Passing the well-manicured lawns of the Jefferson's neighborhood, Don spots a teenager waving them over. Bringing jump kit, oxygen, and monitor-defibrillator, Don and Linda follow Tony into the living room. It is 6:50 P.M.

Ken is vividly aware that two uniformed people are walking toward him with equipment. He feels relief but also embarrassment. He senses his life is out of control. Don and Linda introduce themselves to him and explain they are paramedics. Ken does not understand all they have said. He is aware of the possibly fatal consequences of his illness but fights the idea of death because he has unfinished business—not the paperwork for vacation scheduling but seeing Brenda and Tony through college.

"What seems to be the trouble?" Linda asks.
"My chest."

Don contacts medical control while Linda checks Ken's pulse, respiration, and blood pressure. His pulse is rapid. She palpates for 30 seconds. Don sets up the oxygen. Linda asks Ken how he feels. "It feels like an elephant is sitting on my chest." "Mr. Jefferson, I'm going to give you some oxygen. I have this oxygen mask, which will go over your nose and mouth. It will make it easier for you to breathe."

Don talks with Mrs. Jefferson concerning Mr. Jefferson's recent medical history. He asks her to collect any medications that Ken might be taking.

Don and Linda move him carefully to the stretcher. While setting up the monitor and IV that were ordered, Linda explains that they will be taking him right to the hospital but that they can do some things right here that will make him more comfortable on the way. The rhythm is a sinus tachycardia. She tells Mr. Jefferson that his heart rate is regular but fast.

Janet, Brenda, and Tony watch the EMS providers work intensely on their husband and father. Janet desperately fears losing him. Brenda feels responsible. Tony is worried as well, but he sees his father's bravery in his suffering as heroic. They are all disturbed at the sight of Ken with an oxygen mask and ECG lines in place and an IV line in his arm.

The Jefferson's living room has been transformed into a small emergency department unit by the paramedics and their array of medical equipment. Linda feels Ken's muscles tensing. An almost palpable tension fills the air. She shares with Ken that she senses his anxiety and reassures him that they are doing their best for him.

To the Jefferson family, the movement to the ambulance seems sudden. The abruptness with which Don and Linda begin the transfer catches the family off guard. After a brief discussion, Janet decides to follow with the children. Don tells her they will be going to Memorial Hospital down Winslow Avenue. He reminds them to drive carefully and obey the traffic lights. As Don and Linda head for the ambulance, Ken turns to Janet and says, "Call Jim in the morning. Tell him if I'm in the hospital."

 THE PATIENT'S WORLD

The young or middle-aged heart attack candidate will usually have several risk factors for heart disease.[5] Some risk factors are controllable: a high-fat diet, smoking, obesity, high blood pressure, diabetes. Others such as gender or family history of heart disease are not.[6] Men are more likely than women to have a heart attack in middle age or younger.

The patient's first indications of a heart attack may be chest pain or associated symptoms. Chest pain is a terrifying symptom. The patient may deny the crushing, choking sensation—or deny its significance. "It's only indigestion." "It's only a muscle spasm." "It will go away." The patient may feel embarrassed in calling an ambulance. "Suppose it turns out to be nothing?" The possibility that the symptoms indicate a heart attack is devastating for the patient.

After denial is overcome, a range of concerns associated with a heart attack come to the forefront: job loss; income loss; changes in sexual activity and life style; a generalized concern about "being old." If there is a family history of heart disease, these fears may be compounded by reflections on other relatives with heart problems. The heart attack may not entail any long-term losses, but the patient may envision the bleakest possible future, if he or she survives.

 ## THE BEHAVIOR OF THE PATIENT

Patients may respond to chest pain or chest discomfort in a variety of ways. These responses are summarized in Box 2–1. Three of these responses increase the patient's risk and may complicate your treatment of the patient as well. As noted previously, denial can lead a patient to hide symptoms from family and EMS providers. A patient who responds by isolation may hide (perhaps in a bathroom or a bedroom). A patient who challenges symptoms may try to work through the pain by engaging in strenuous activity. Recognition, though, can lead to appropriate help-seeking behavior.

Managed care organizations may require their patients to seek advice before calling EMS. A patient with heart attack symptoms is an exception to this rule, but patients who call EMS (or whose family calls) may be anxious about their health care coverage.

Very often the first reaction is to wait and see: "It will go away." This may be demonstrated by behavior designed to ignore the pain or by ineffective measures to relieve it. These efforts may persist even when the patient's discomfort is obvious to family and friends. If it is **angina,** the pain will go away with rest, usually within 10 minutes; pain from myocardial infarction will not. At its most severe, the patient will be helpless, in the grip of a crushing pain that prevents activity.[3]

BOX 2–1

BEHAVIORAL RESPONSES TO CHEST PAIN

Denial	Stoically holding on
Isolation	Hiding from others
Challenge	Increasing activity to "work through the pain"
Recognition	Seeking help

THE EMOTIONS AND THOUGHTS BEHIND THE BEHAVIOR

Understanding the chest pain patient's thought process and emotional response can increase your empathy and your effectiveness. Typically the patient's thoughts focus around the three D's: denial, devastation, death. The dominant emotion is anxiety. Denial can include either rationalization or minimization. The patient holds out hope—mentally—that the pain is not significant. For example, "It's indigestion" or "This is nothing to worry about, whatever it is." The patient may focus on anything except the heart. Ken focuses on his work schedules.

The devastation phase follows when mental or physical efforts to relieve pain have failed. For most patients, the principal affect is anxiety. Anxiety, in contrast to fear, is **free-floating.** It is not associated with a particular object. It may result in panic. In the devastation phase, thoughts turn to unfinished business, obligations not met. The patient fears that everything will change: job, sex life, physical activities. The actual extent of cardiac damage and impairment in physical functioning will vary tremendously, but the belief that the experience is devastating is almost universal.

Finally, anxiety about—even expectation of—death may become dominant. Everyone knows people who have died of heart attacks. The patient may even believe—mistakenly—that a heart attack is inevitably fatal. Facing eternity, recognizing one's own mortality—perhaps for the first time—casts a distinctive stamp on future activities and relationships. Every survivor's perspective on life changes after a heart attack. Ken looks at the bleak future his family will have if he is permanently disabled or absent.

 FAMILY/BYSTANDER RESPONSES

Your obligation is to the patient in distress, but the family is also in need of help. Family members also experience anxiety and guilt. Janet senses Ken's worsening condition. She may blame herself for not correcting Ken's bad habits or for not having been more supportive. Even more important, she may blame herself for not calling for help sooner. Brenda feels guilty: she believes the stress she created brought on the heart attack. Neither attitude is healthy for the family members. To the extent that Ken's current level of anxiety is affected by those around him, it may be unhealthy for him as well. Beliefs about responsibility can devastate survivors if the patient dies. Tony's response—fleeing from the scene and waiting for the ambulance in the front yard—at least had the advantage of guiding the responders to the right address.

In our scenario, the family members did not act constructively. There are two family responses that can harm the patient. First, the family may support the patient's denial, delaying help. Second, at the other extreme, they may feel that the heart attack is "the end" and may begin to psychologically withdraw from the patient even before help arrives. Citizen cardiopulmonary resuscitation (CPR) instruction is important not only because of the life-saving skills that are taught but for the CHD education they learn at the same time.

Many families will respond with love and concern to a family member having chest pain. They may recognize the urgency of the situation and call for help. However, you are in an excellent position to assess family and bystander behavior and emotions and to provide some on-scene education of the patient and the family.

 ## PROVIDER RESPONSES

Generally, EMS teams respond effectively to patients with chest pain. However, these situations do cause anxiety. Responders who have seen a patient go into cardiac arrest in the ambulance may be more likely to experience such anxiety. One possible danger is that you may take unwarranted risks in trying to reach the patient quickly.

 ## INTERVENTION STRATEGIES

Observe

The potential seriousness of the patient's condition does not allow for a casual walk about or a chat with friends or relatives. However, do not drive carelessly or run recklessly into the scene. Hidden obstacles such as toys or garden tools can pose a threat to your safety. In sizing up the scene, look out for potential hazards and plan access to the patient. Plan your exit carefully as well.

Consider the patient's physical condition and emotional state. You cannot assume that chest pain in an older man is necessarily a symptom of acute myocardial infarction, nor can you assume that chest pain in a young man or woman is not, although other explanations may be more likely.[4]

Interact

You can reduce anxiety by the way in which you approach the patient. The chest pain patient requires a confident, rapid response. Your style of address, posture, and position may be more important than your spoken words. People under stress will pick up more from your tone than your actual statements. Linda and Don move smoothly as a team, presenting a model of coordination and efficiency. They introduced themselves, but began their assessment promptly once they established a relationship with Ken. They also asked the right questions, saving precious time. They explained what they were doing. Advanced Life Support is a mystery to the general public despite wide exposure on the news and reality TV. Even basic procedures can be confusing to a patient who expects the ambulance to "load and go." Universal precautions against infectious disease and risk management procedures can also be disturbing to patients.

You can help families and patients to understand and manage their anxiety and guilt by following the suggestions given here. These actions will reduce family tensions now and during the hospitalization and recovery period.

Ask

When possible, make your initial questions open-ended. That is, questions should call for an explanation by the patient rather than for a simple "yes" or "no" response. For instance, "What seems to be the trouble?" is a better opening than "Does your chest hurt?" The open-ended question allows for a more detailed assessment of the patient's level of consciousness and organization of thought. It also minimizes the possibility that a patient will give an answer he thinks you expect. The OPQRST method of questioning, shown in Box 2–2, fits nicely with an open-ended approach.

Taking a SAMPLE history is important because it will affect the patient's awareness of or concern about his current condition. It may also prompt the patient to recall a similar event from the past and will enable him to relate the current event to past ones. Box 2–3 provides SAMPLE questions pertinent to the patient with a cardiac emergency.

Act

Your teamwork and coordination will demonstrate your professionalism to the patient. If you improvise or muddle through, you send an unwanted message. If you have your roles and responsibilities worked out in advance, you not only provide better care, but you increase the patient's confidence in the care you are providing.

BOX 2–2

THE OPQRST METHOD OF ASKING ABOUT PAIN

Onset	When did these symptoms begin?
Provocation	What brought on (or provoked) the pain? Does anything seem to help?
Quality	How does the pain feel (e.g., sharp, dull, squeezing)?
Region	Where do you feel this pain?
Radiation	Does the discomfort go anywhere else?
Relief	Is there anything that seems to offer relief of the symptoms?
Severity	On a scale of 1 to 10, with 10 being the worst pain you've ever had, how would you rate this pain?
Timing	When did the pain begin? Is it constant?

BOX 2–3

SAMPLE HISTORY QUESTIONS FOR THE CARDIAC PATIENT

Symptoms	Ask the patient about the symptoms he is experiencing. Ask the patient to rate the pain on a pain scale. Ask how long he has been experiencing these symptoms.
Allergies	Ask the patient if he has any allergies. Specifically ask about medication allergies.
Medications	Ask the patient if he is taking any medications. Medications related to hypertension or a heart disorder may offer clues to a possible preexisting condition. Be sure to ask about over-the-counter medications and diet or herbal supplements as well.
Past Medical History	Ask the patient about any prior episodes of a similar nature. Was he able to do anything that offered relief at that time?
Last Oral Intake	Ask the patient about what he has eaten recently or if he has Intake taken anything to relieve the pain.
Events Leading up to Current Event	Ask the patient about his activity prior to feeling the pain.

Confidence, care, and control also serve to reassure the family and other bystanders. They struggle with anxieties similar to those of the patient, but they also have the time to watch. That time can appear to stretch on endlessly. Explaining your actions and giving the family and patient a time frame can reduce anxiety. To Tony, who only knew that his father had a pain in the chest, it seemed unbelievable that the paramedics were putting a needle in his father's arm. To Janet, who expected the team to rush to the hospital, the delay was confusing.

Attend

Linda and Don were busy with initial (and subsequent) vital signs, setting up and reading the monitor, setting up oxygen, and starting an IV. A patient, such as Ken, may show increasing agitation, not only in the content of his speech, but in tone of voice and body language. Taking stock of these changes and offering specific appropriate reassurance is important.

Document

Documentation issues are straightforward. Document all response and transport times. Take vital signs and record them regularly. The OPQRST approach described in Box 2–2 is a good guide in describing the patient's complaint in your report.

 ## CONSIDERATIONS FOR EMS PROVIDERS

You will feel strong emotions as you work with patients in pain and with potentially life-threatening conditions. If you do not handle these emotions well, you may build up undesirable defenses. These include developing a protective **delusion** of invincibility; retreating into a cold, technical approach to patients; inability to function, or a sarcastic manner that distances you from your patient's experiences. These defenses may succeed in the short run, but they fail in the long run. The sad fact is that these defenses can result in the development of serious pathologies.

The delusion of invincibility is often seen in addicted health care providers who witness the ravages of alcohol and other drugs but continue to drink to intoxication on a regular basis or claim to be able to handle their excesses because they have seen what drugs can do. However, EMS providers can also deny their risk of heart disease by ignoring the standard advice on smoking, diet, and moderation in alcohol use that is recommended by public health experts.

An EMS provider who makes technical efficiency the end rather than the means in patient care exhibits a cold, technical approach. Efficiency and team work are essential, but good interpersonal skills such as making eye contact and listening empathically must also be part of the care.

An inability to function or freezing at the scene may relate to early professional experiences or even to personal experiences prior to becoming involved with EMS. For example, after her patient went into cardiac arrest in the ambulance on one of her first runs, one EMS provider described how she became panic stricken when the dispatcher announced a "possible heart attack."

The gallows humor defense is less destructive than the previous three, but it can lead to a callousness and lack of concern for the patient as a person, unless it is balanced with a sincere ventilation of feelings. Humor can ease the anger, frustration, and grief and serve an important healing function. To laugh at yourself, and with your colleagues, and your patients can be therapeutic, as well as providing a good situation for learning. The danger arises when the humor focuses on put-downs and disrespectful observations.

If you see these reactions in yourself or your partner, take action. We recommend some specific possibilities in Chapter 16.

CONCLUSION

Teamwork is essential in caring for a cardiac patient. A confident, competent team will provide state-of-the-art medical care and will demonstrate confidence in working with each other.

REVIEW QUESTIONS

1. List at least three risk factors for heart disease.
2. List three behaviors that can be dangerous to a person with chest pain.
3. Why may family members of a patient with chest pain experience anxiety and guilt?
4. Why are open-ended questions better than closed-ended questions?
5. What do the initials OPQRST mean in assessment? Can you think of some other situations besides chest pain where this approach might be useful?
6. What are some of the reactions that EMS providers might develop that suggest that they are having problems in caring for their patients?

EXERCISES

1. Think about the people you know who have been diagnosed with CHD. How did the diagnosis affect their lifestyle?
2. Do you know people with serious or life-threatening conditions? Did they go for medical help as soon as they became aware that something was wrong? Did they minimize the early symptoms?
3. Families can help or hinder your care of the patient. What ways do you think they might help or hinder you in caring for a cardiac patient?
4. Role play a situation with a patient with chest pain. How would you and your partner share responsibilities?
5. What aspects of the emergency care of the patient with a myocardial infarction might be disturbing to the patient and the family?

REFERENCES

1. www.nhlbi.nih.gov/health/public/other/chdfacts.htm
2. Emery, C. F., & Becker, N. L. (1998). "Psychosocial issues and the heart" in E. J. Topol, Ed., *Cardiovascular Medicine* (pp. 249–262). Philadelphia: Lippincott-Raven.

3. Halberstam, M., & Lesher, S. (1976) *A coronary event* (p. 25). Philadelphia: JB Lippincott.

4. Dernocoeur, K. (1996). *Streetsense: communication, safety, and control* (3rd ed.). Bowie, MD: Creative Options.

5. Mazeika, P. (2001). Aborted sudden cardiac death: A clinical perspective. *Postgrad Med. J. 77* (908), 363–370.

6. Criss, E. (1997). An unrecognized epidemic: woman and heart disease. *Journal of Emergency Medical Services, 22* (5), 58–63, 1997.

FURTHER INFORMATION

Internet Resources

American Heart Association: www.americanheart.org

Media Resources

Books

Lewis, K., & Handal, K. (2001). *Sensible analysis of the ECG.* Clifton Park, NY: Delmar Learning.

Fuster, V., Alexandre, R. W., & O'Rourke, R. A. (2001). *Hurst's the heart* (10th ed.). New York: McGraw-Hill Professional Publishing.

Myers, J. W. (2000). *Automated defibrillation for professional and lay rescuers.* Clifton Park, NY: Delmar Learning.

Rath, M. (1997). *Why animals don't get heart attacks but people do.* Sunnyvale, CA: Matthias Rath Inc.

CHAPTER 3

The Elderly

Handle with Care

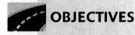

OBJECTIVES

Upon completion of this chapter, you should be able to:

- Understand the significance of the elderly population both in our society and in your work.
- Understand the medical and psychological issues that may arise when dealing with the elderly.
- Outline the normal process of aging and thus be able to differentiate that from the effects of disease.
- Demonstrate how to gear your intervention to the elder patients' and their families' realities, fears and hopes.

THE CHALLENGE

Never before have there been more elderly and never before have the seniors been more healthy—yes, healthy seniors. In 1997, there were 20 million women and 14 million men over 65 years old. The percentage of the American population over 65 years old continues to soar: in 1940, it was 9 percent; by 2000, 13 percent; and by 2030 it will be 21 percent (Box 3–1). It is estimated that by 2030, there will be 69.4 million senior Americans![1] Contrary to popular belief, only 5 percent of the current senior population is in nursing facilities.[2]

Although the majority of the elderly are living in their communities, they are vulnerable to many health problems. EMS providers will experience an increase in involvement with senior citizens in the coming years. In the intersection of their health emergencies and your interventions lies the critical and delicate balance between their and your needs and fascinating care paradoxes.

BOX 3-1

SCOPE

By 2023 20 percent of all people in the United States will be 65 and over! This population constitutes a major part of your work.[1]

They want and need help but they want to maintain their independence. They have long medical histories but also many current strengths. They are alone and yet they often have a remarkable support network. EMS interventions must address their problems while considering their capabilities. A swift response may be necessary but the elderly require a certain amount of time and patience (Box 3–2).

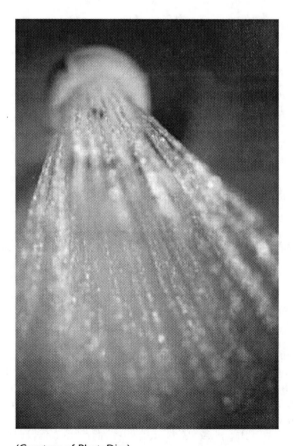

(Courtesy of PhotoDisc)

THE PATIENT AND THE SITUATION

Burt Williamson, age 79, has fallen in the shower. He cannot get up. His legs are weak, his balance is poor, and his blood pressure is **labile**. He feels embarrassed, frustrated, and overwhelmed. His family doctor had suggested he use a walker in the shower, but he thought he could at least shower without assistance. Now a little voice in his head calls him a fool.

His wife of 56 years, Paula, has back trouble and knows she cannot lift him. She feels desperate and scared. She also wants to say to Burt, "I told you so," but dares not say it. Both Burt and Paula fear that this event will make their daughter, Julia, and son, Burt Junior, demand that they move into an elderly housing unit or nursing facility. They fear such a move not only as their loss of independence but also as the kiss of death.

Paula reluctantly calls 911.

The scene shifts to the Public Safety Center, where veteran EMS providers Susie Hale and Big Mike Bolton receive the call. Although they are quick to get into the vehicle, they do not feel the rush of cardiac or respiratory arrest urgency.

However, Mike has a mental flash of his grandparents and suddenly feels very protective of the couple they are about to help. He accelerates. Sue, runs a mental check list of all the possible causes for a fall and a subsequent inability to get up. She wonders if the gentleman could have had a stroke or heart attack or **syncope** episode? Or perhaps he has had a medication reaction or interaction. Maybe he is diabetic?

They arrive at the home and Mike, grabbing the emergency kit, heads for the door. Paula Williamson opens the door and just stands there. Her blank expression speaks volumes. Finally, she, in frustration and shock, points to the first-floor bathroom. As Mike speeds past her, he mentally chastises himself for not introducing himself to Mrs. Williamson, and he heads for the bathroom.

Burt is lying on the tiled floor, looking up with alarm and embarrassment. His first utterance is, "Please, give me a towel." Silently, Mike feels relieved that

BOX 3–2

SIGNIFICANCE FOR EMS

The growing senior population presents with a vast array of physical and emotional problems. It constitutes a group at risk and represents a major EMS responsibility.

at least Mr. Burt Williamson is *with it!* He is oriented to the situation and thus he has passed the mental status examination. Mike helps Mr. Williamson get covered with a towel as Susie and Mrs. Williamson appear outside the bathroom door. Mrs. Williamson remains quiet and fearful.

Susie tells Mr. Williamson she is first going to take his blood pressure. As she does so, she realizes that she has actually been yelling at him. Paula announces, "He has fallen but he's not hard of hearing." After taking the pressure and finding it to be 138/94, she finds and then checks his pulse and observes his respirations.

With his vital signs stable and not emergent, Mike starts to ask what seems to Burt and Paula a lot of medical questions. He asks about any recent trauma, medical illnesses, medications, and stresses. Burt begins to answer with a "see here, young man" attitude. Although the Williamsons are relieved by the response, they are also sensing this is not a medical emergency and that the EMS providers are "just kids."

Their ire is further provoked when Susie asks both to see Burt's medication and to look in the medicine cabinet. They are somewhat placated by Susie's request to call Burt's doctor. Finally, with Mike and Susie on either side of Burt, he slowly and gratefully gets to his feet. They help him to a chair. After checking Burt's blood pressure and pulse again, Mike suggests that the patient drink some fluids and rest. He also recommends that a walker be used in the shower. Neither Susie nor Mike think he should be taken to the hospital.

Burt and Paula are both relieved and annoyed by this nontransport solution. They are glad the fall was not too serious but frustrated that they could not solve it themselves. Mike and Susie complete their forms and they, too, feel both successful and annoyed by this run. They did help—great! Yet, what they did, did not require all their skills and training.

 THE PATIENT'S WORLD

The elderly live in a world of fascinating contradictions and contrasts. On the one hand their world is expanding yet on the other hand it is contracting. In this period in their lives seniors have more time to spend on activities they enjoy and are able explore new activities; however, they often feel as if time is running out to do all they want to do. New technologies and research are allowing people to live longer but the fear of a life-altering illness or injury is ever present. They have family and friends yet their family and friends are getting sick and dying. Independence is highly valued while at the same time the elderly appreciate their need for help.

The world of retirement provides a wide range of activities, including returning to school, taking courses, and traveling. It also encompasses a very wide spectrum of volunteering opportunities; for example, in libraries, schools, hospitals, hospice, museums, and community projects. Many retirees also choose to explore employment possibilities ranging from the supermarket to Wal-Mart and day care to consulting.

As people get older they are particularly conscious of their own limitations. Yes, there are more opportunities, but they are very selective as to how to invest their time. For example, many seniors recognize their difficulty in nighttime driving; therefore, they restrict their travel and courses to the daylight hours. They may hike but appreciate that their trips will be shorter than they were when they were younger. The natural process of aging called **senescence** results in seniors' sensory limitations in hearing, vision, smelling, touching, and tasting (see Box 3–3).

The issue of time offers yet another example of elder paradoxes. Once retired, they often seem to have more time available. Yet, many of the elderly report that they are busier since they left their job than ever before. In fact, one retiree facetiously noted that she did not know how she ever had time for her job! Most seniors are aware of time limits of their lives and their own death.

People are living longer and healthier than ever before. The statistics show their increased longevity and demonstrate better health in general than any previous generation. Yet, aging does bring health problems and chronic illnesses. Aging means hardening of the arteries, brittle bones, decreased immune system responsiveness, and loss of skin elasticity. Many elderly take multiple prescriptions and over-the-counter medications. Seniors are both healthy and frail.

Despite the image of the lonely elder person, most are gregarious and have family and friends. They are engaged in many social and community group events and activities. Yet, they are also painfully aware of the health status and longevity of their family and friends. Many seniors commence their day by reading the obituaries of their local newspaper.

Finally, as the New Hampshire state license plate proclaims—Live Free or Die—most of the elderly demand, fight for, and cling to their independence. They personify the John Wayne image. They want to remain in the community and be involved or to be left alone—either way—*on their own terms. In fact, 95 percent of people over 65 years old live in the community* (Figure 3–1).[1] However, as they grow older, most grow wiser and appreciate their need for assistance. The elderly do go to doctors when indicated; they accept visiting nurses and home help; and they will go to day-care programs. But they also want and demand their *dignity*.

 ## THE BEHAVIOR OF THE PATIENT

Discussing elder behavior highlights a significant conflict. There are many changes with aging called senescence; however, by focusing on them and overgeneralizing based on them you run the risk of stereotyping the elder population. This can imply prejudice against the elderly called **ageism.** Accepting this fine line, a number of behaviors remain that must be appreciated when working with the elderly. Such behaviors include deliberate movements, slower

BOX 3-3

SENESCENCE—THE BIOLOGY OF THE AGING PROCESS

Cardiovascular System

- blood pressure increases
- heart rate decreases
- progression of arteriosclerosis
- cardiac output decreases with activity
- heart valves become more rigid, which can compromise cardiac function
- may exhibit arrhythmias

Endocrine System

- thyroid functions remain intact
- decrease in ability to metabolize glucose
- decreased production of estrogen and testosterone

Gastrointestinal System

- decreased hydrochloric acid (HCl) secretion in the stomach
- decreased small bowel absorption
- diminished liver biodegrading process resulting in longer drug half-lives
- loss of teeth makes eating difficult

Reproductive System

- women experience menopause
- men in their 70s and 80s experience a decline in sperm production

Immune System

- decrease in some immune cells
- decline in T and B cell responsiveness
- infections more likely to be fatal due to decreased response

Integumentary System

- the skin wrinkles and thins
- more malignances
- the nails thicken and easily split
- brown, pigmented areas develop on the hands, arms, and face

Musculoskeletal System

- decrease of muscle mass from approximately 80 percent to 35 percent
- increase in muscle and joint aches
- demineralization leading to more fractures

BOX 3–3 CONTINUED

Nervous System

- decrease in gray matter
- increase in cerebral spinal fluid
- in the very old the brain may decrease in size and weight

The Senses

- Hearing, presbycusis (hearing loss with age), decrease in high-frequency appreciation
- Smell, decrease in aroma sensitivity
- Taste, decrease in taste sensations
- Touch, decrease in touch sensatory ability
- Vision, cataracts develop; presbyopia (diminished visual acuity with age)

Respiratory System

- decrease in respiratory functions

Urinary System

- decrease in all renal functions including **erythropoietin** (the hormone that triggers red blood cell production) leading to anemia

Adapted from information from Leventhal, E. A. (1996). Biology of aging. In J. Sadavoy, L. W. Lazarus, L. F. Jarvik, & G. T. Grossberg, Eds. *Comprehensive review of geriatric psychiatry—II* (2nd ed., pp. 81–112). Washington, D.C.: American Psychiatric Press.)

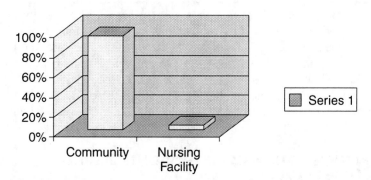

Where Seniors Live

FIGURE 3–1 The majority of the elderly remain living in their own homes and as active members of the community well into old age.[1]

response times, gait instability, a shift in sleep patterns, and diminished appetite. Within the elderly population there is an increase in the rate of suicides. In 1997, men and women over age 65 made up 13 percent of the U.S. population. However, they accounted for 19 percent of all suicides. The suicide rate for white men age 85 or older is six times the national average.[3] Seniors make more visits to health-care providers. Also a large number of elderly live alone.

Perhaps the most notable feature of aging is that the elderly act more deliberately. They consider their acts and actions. As a result, they simply do things at a slower rate. Such behavior is often the source of many jokes about being stuck behind some older driver on the highway or shopping behind an elder in the supermarket. Simply put, seniors move more slowly and require more time than younger folks to do many things.

In that same vein, seniors have a slower reaction time. It takes them longer to process material and to respond to it. However, that does not mean they are necessarily poorer drivers than younger ones. They often are better at anticipating situations and therefore avoiding them.

With age comes gait instability. The elderly may become unsure of their footing and experience falls. As a result of more brittle bones, they are more susceptible to fractures.

With age, people experience a shift in their sleep patterns. They retire earlier, and, more importantly, they get up earlier. They require less nighttime sleep. For many, the early awakening is perceived as a problem.

With age, many elders simply eat less. This change in eating behavior may reflect their diminished number of taste buds or that they live alone and therefore often eat alone. Decreased appetite can lead to weight loss.

The suicide rate dramatically increases with age.[1] The incidence of clinical depression accelerates in the elderly. Loss represents the critical dynamic that causes depression, and with aging there are many losses.

The elderly see their physicians and visit health-care providers more frequently than do younger people, reflecting their increased number of health problems. Doctor visits have become a routine in the lives of many elderly people.

Finally, many elders live alone, and this number has increased over the years. For the age group 65–74, in 1970, 11.3 percent of men and 31.6 percent of women lived alone. In 1995 14 percent of men and 32 percent of women lived alone. However, if you look at the population that is older than 75 years, in 1970 19.1 percent of men and 37 percent of women lived alone. By the end of the 20th century, approximately 23 percent of men and 53 percent of women lived alone.[1]

THE EMOTIONS AND THOUGHTS BEHIND THE BEHAVIOR

There are three emotions and thoughts that represent abnormality in the aging population. Of interest, these three—*depression, memory loss, and fatigue*—which constitute indicators of serious psychiatric or medical problems, are often mistaken for a normal facet of aging.

We often hear the expression *a depressed old man or woman*. It is often uttered as if this were the expected and normal state of affairs for the elderly. True, there can be a sadness in elders reflecting a number of accrued losses that inevitability accompany growing older, but this is not clinical depression. Major depression according to the American Psychiatric Association's diagnostic criteria (DSM IV) consists of daily sadness, every day disruptions of sleep (**insomnia** or **hypersomnia**), decreased or increased appetite every day, daily psychomotor agitation or retardation, with either preoccupation with death or suicidal ideation and impairment in social and vocational functions over a prolonged period.[4]

If the elderly do meet these criteria, then they are depressed and *that depression can be and must be treated*. Rephrased, depression in the elderly is not normal. Depression represents a pathological condition but it does respond to treatment.

Perhaps, one of the most common statements you hear when someone forgets something is, "I just had a senior moment!" Thus, it comes as quite a surprise to many that memory loss is *not* a normal part of aging. Certainly, name retrieval is more difficult with aging, and processing new information takes longer with growing older. Yet, recent and immediate memory loss are not regular facets of aging. Nor is being disoriented to time, place, and person part of the normal aging process. Therefore, if the person demonstrates inability to recall immediate information and recent events and shows evidence of disorientation, look at **dementia** or **delirium** as possible causes.[5] When a 79-year-old gentleman goes out for a package of cigarettes at night, gets lost, and is returned by the local police, think Alzheimer's and not a senior moment.

Seniors often tire more easily than do younger folks. Some prefer an afternoon nap. Tiring more easily is part of aging. However, when an elder person complains of fatigue, think medical illnesses. Exhaustion represents an abnormal condition. A host of diseases present as fatigue, including anemia, heart failure, infections, breathing disorders, and cancer.[6]

 ## FAMILY/BYSTANDER RESPONSES

For the families of the elderly there emerge a host of contrasting thoughts and feelings. They see the gradual decline of their loved one but at the same time want to provide companionship and love. They find frailty yet they also discover wisdom in the elderly. Paula wants her husband to get better but she does not want to be alone. Families appreciate the wonders of medicine yet fear change and worry about side effects. Like Paula they see others as attempting both to help and *control* them. Thus, families mourn the losses and celebrate the relationships. For example, one daughter and her family cared for her mother who had Alzheimer's. They saw the mother gradually decline and were sad about it. Yet, they took solace and joy in the moments when the mother was **lucid**.

PROVIDER RESPONSES

EMS provider responses to the elderly can often run to two extremes as Susie Hale and Big Mike Bolton have demonstrated. On the one hand Susie suggests the cynical view of aging. Cynics see the elderly as out of date, useless, and in the way. They make fun of the way seniors dress and act. Their attitudes reflect a sense of intolerance and often annoyance. One of the authors taught a course on aging. Several of the nursing students had the most insensitive things to say about the elderly. One admonished her classmates to avoid shopping at the supermarket on Thursday morning. That is when the seniors shop and "they are so slow!"

On the other hand, like Mike, many take a patronizing view of the elderly. They want to help them and tell them what to do. Although seeing seniors in the image of your parents and grandparents may suggest compassion and empathy, it also can lead to intrusions into their sovereignty and independence.

The best response involves both a healthy respect for the elderly and an appreciation of their strengths and weaknesses.

INTERVENTION STRATEGIES

Observe

EMS providers are in a pivotal position when assessing a senior citizen to make some critical observations not only about that person but also his environment and his support system.

When they first see the person, they can make a number of determinations of physical and mental status. Certainly, just a handshake offers a clue about that individual's circulation as well as his temperature. The attire may reveal many clues about his hygiene and ability to care for himself. For example, a dirty shirt with numerous burn holes suggests possibilities of dementia. Tears may reflect depression. Observing that person's ambulating shows how stable he is. A quick mental status evaluation, inquiring about the date, the place, and the person as well as immediate, recent, and distant recall, provide critical information for determining the possibility of delirium or dementia.

Furthermore, EMS providers observe self-destructive threats, suicide notes, or suicidal behavior that must be responded to. Additionally, just being in the home gives EMS providers the opportunity to review the medications by a quick survey of the medicine cabinet for both prescription and over-the-counter drugs. (It is often amazing that people do not realize all the medications they are taking, and they often do not report them all to their physicians.)

Beyond the person, EMS providers can assess the environment. Things such as gas stoves left on, mice or rats running about, no heat in the winter or excessive heat in the summer, burned pans, mountains of garbage, or empty refrigerators suggest that the patient is an **elder at risk.** This term designates a category of problem that requires further assessment and possibly some sort of intervention. Most states have programs to respond to elders at risk. Some states have adult protective workers. In either case, a trained staff member, often working under contract to the state government, is empowered to visit the elder's home.

In addition, EMS providers are in a good position to observe the relationship between the patient and others. That interaction can reveal a variety of key dynamics. Sometimes, the caregivers may be treating the senior very well. In other situations, they can be inflicting harm on him or simply not feeding him well (negligence). Such treatment is elder abuse and requires a reporting process to initiate interventions to protect that individual from any further harm. In other instances, the senior may be inflicting harm on his caregivers. In one case, EMS providers discovered a 69-year-old man with chronic obstructive pulmonary disease (COPD) who had been beating his wife. Besides addressing the patient's pulmonary problem, they also had to secure protection for his wife.

Interact

The interaction between the elderly and EMS providers must follow a number of key principles. The communication must be done respectfully, directly, clearly, with a deliberate **cadence,** and with anticipatory explanations.

First and foremost, many health-care providers have a tendency to treat the elderly both in a patronizing manner and to subtly make fun of them. This behavior can be exhibited by EMS providers who call elder patients, whom they do not know, by the patient's first name. Too frequently, EMS providers say, "Joey, come over here" or "sit down here, honey." Call elders by their full names with the dignity of the appropriate title of Mister or Miss or Mrs.

The elderly want direct and clear information. They often object to **euphemisms**. An elderly gentleman suffered a fatal heart attack at home. The team responded quickly and professionally. Yet, throughout the resuscitation they recognized the futility of the procedure, and wanted to transport him to the hospital. They told his wife of the plan and offered vague answers to her questions. Then, she said, "He's dead, isn't he?" The point is that the elderly have been around for a long time and appreciate candid information. They not only do not like "bull" but will also tell you that they don't!

When speaking with these folks, EMS providers will be most effective if they adopt and develop a slow deliberate **cadence,** which means speaking in a clear, unhurried, not quiet but not shouting voice. This communication style incorporates the reality that the elderly require time to comprehend new material and may have hearing problems.

Finally, the elder, as with all patients, needs and appreciates knowing what will happen next and the reason for it. If you are going to transport the patient to the hospital, tell the patient and the family of the trip and the rationale for it. Then, as you proceed in the intervention, repeat your plan. This type of preparation avoids making assumptions of what they know and what they expect.

Ask

You must ask many questions about the health of the elderly, their medical care, and their lifestyle. As noted earlier, elders often have a long list of medical problems. And those diagnoses frequently translate into a significant variety of medications. In addition, if a person lives long enough, his or her history has a higher possibility of surgical events. Finally, some elders have a less-than-complete diet; therefore, an inquiry into dietary habits is in order.

So, to ask or not to ask, is not the question. The key issue remains how to ask. Again, as with all patients, the tone must be to secure information for their benefit not to be accusatory. Hence, a very quick explanation as to the usefulness of the question helps to deflect the "attack" quality of the question. Here, EMS providers need mental status information to assess dementia and delirium as well as suicidal and homicidal intent. So ask, but do so respectfully, preserving the patient's and the family's dignity.

Act

As with any patient, it is very important to announce and explain your actions in advance. However, elderly patients may benefit from repeated explanations as you proceed. Abrupt, uninformed moves can be a source of further discomfort to the patient and family. Actions should be smooth and well orchestrated.

Attend

There are several reasons why senior patients should not be left alone. First, an unattended elderly person in a moment of confusion (dementia or delirium) may sustain additional injury. In one case, an 80-year-old man, complaining of chest discomfort, was left alone on the gurney. He was experiencing some disorientation and memory impairment. As he tried to get up to get some water, he fell from the stretcher and fractured his left femur. Second, the medical problem generating the emergency requires close monitoring. Third, medical intervention and transport is anxiety provoking for many elderly patients. Therefore, having personnel stay with the patient can be reassuring and comforting for that patient.

Attending to the patient can also mean attending to the patient's property. When transporting a patient, make sure that you take the time to lock up the home. Ask the elder patient if he would like you to contact family members (sons, daughters, or grandchildren) or a neighbor. Elderly patients may also have pets. Pets are sometimes the only companion the patient has and the patient may be very concerned for the care of the pet if he needs to go to the hospital. This pet issue must be dealt with.

Document

As in all medical assessments and interventions, documentation represents a critical aspect of care; however, for the elderly it can be even more important. For example, the elder patient's vital signs not only constitute valuable assessment clues but also can be used to compare with previously recorded material. Many of the elderly have extensive medical records. Hence, most of them will have baseline data to look at.

In addition, EMS providers must be particularly careful to record only objective medical material. Words such as cantankerous, spinster, senile old codger, reclusive, or secluded should not be used. They only reflect your prejudices and not clinical information. Box 3–4 summarizes and EMS providers intervention strategies.

 CONSIDERATIONS FOR EMS PROVIDERS

In the final analysis, EMS providers deal with a host of often contradictory feelings and reactions in working with the elderly. Their responses range from priorities and system concerns to family and personal issues. So as a group and as individuals, EMS providers confront an interesting array of emotions.

BOX 3–4

SUMMARY OF STRATEGY

Observe	appearance, where and *how* the person lives
Interact	slowly, with careful explanations
Ask	clearly state the questions
Act	inform people before doing anything; explain the intervention
Attend	stay with the patient
Document	record times, interventions, medications

On the system level, EMS providers acknowledge that the elderly represent a significant number of calls. Yet, they also recognize that these responses can take a long time and some may even be unnecessary. If Burt Williamson had accepted the idea of a walker in the shower, EMS would not have needed to be called.

The family issues often involve feelings about the EMS providers' parents and grandparents. "How would they like their loved ones to be responded to?" does go through the EMS providers' minds. Many want to help those older folks; some resent it. Finally, working with the elderly forces all EMS providers to confront their own future frailty, dependence, and mortality.

CONCLUSION

Perhaps, EMS providers can learn some successful life strategies from what they witness in the elderly. Many seniors live long, productive lives based on exercise, diet, and stress control. Chapter 16 discusses life health strategies for EMS providers. Many of the elderly can also teach us how to live longer and better.

REVIEW QUESTIONS

1. Why is the aging of the American population significant to EMS providers?
2. Define senescence. What kinds of physical changes are related to senescence?
3. What signs of illness or deterioration, often considered part of the normal aging process, may indicate significant medical conditions?
4. What is ageism and how might it be manifested in your work?

EXERCISES

1. Invite one or several senior citizens to talk to your group about their lives, their work, their families, their hopes, and their fears as well as their medical experiences. Ask them about their medical emergency experiences.
2. Visit either a senior center or retirement community and observe active, healthy senior citizens.
3. Visit a nursing facility and observe the special techniques used with ill elderly residents and those with Alzheimer's disease.
4. As a group, discuss your feelings about getting old. Discuss the care you expect and demand for your parents and grandparents.

5. How would you gear your intervention knowing that you were going to be assisting an elderly person?

REFERENCES

1. Vander Zanden, J. W. (2000). *Human development* (7th ed.). Boston: McGraw Hill.
2. Moody, H. R. (2000). *Aging: concepts and controversies* (3rd ed.). Thousand Oaks, CA: Pine Forge Press.
3. Older Adults: Depression and Suicide Facts. http://www.nimh.gov/publicat/elderlydepsuicide.cfm.
4. American Psychiatric Association. (1994). *Diagnostic and statistical manual of mental disorders* (4th ed.). Washington, DC: Author.
5. Reisberg, B. (1996). Alzheimer's disease. In J. Sadavoy, L. W. Lazarus, L. F. Jarvik, & G. T. Grossberg, Eds. *Comprehensive review of geriatric psychiatry–II* (2nd ed., pp. 401–458). Washington, DC: American Psychiatric Press.
6. Braunwald, E., Fauci, A. S., Kasper, D. L., Hauser, S. L., Longo, D. L., & Jameson, J. L. (2001). *Harrison's principles of internal medicine* (15th ed.). New York: McGraw-Hill.

FURTHER INFORMATION

Internet Resources

Administration on Aging: www.aoa.dhhs.gov

Alzheimer's Association: www.alz.org

American Association of Homes and Services for the Aging: www.aahsa.org

American Society on Aging: www.asaging.org

Bureau of the Census: www.census.gov

Center for Disease Control and Prevention: www.cdc.gov

Healthgate: www.healthgate.com

Merck Manual, which includes Merck Manual of Geriatrics: www.merck.com

National Institute on Aging: www.nih.gov/nia/

National Institutes of Health: www.nih.gov/health

Older Adults: Depression and Suicide Facts: http://www.nimh.gov/publicat/elderlydepsuicide.cfm

Media Resources

Movies

On Golden Pond

Grumpy Old Men (One and Two)

Books and Articles

Dollemore, D. & the editors of Prevention. (2001). *Seniors guide to pain-free living*. New York: St. Martin Press.

Downs, H. (1994). *Fifty to forever*. Nashville, TN: Thomas Nelson Publishers.

Harvard Medical School family health guide. (1999). New York: Simon and Schuster.

Henderson, C. (1997). *Funny, I don't feel old! How to flourish after fifty*. Oakland, CA: ICS Press.

Hodgson, H. (1995). *Alzheimer's: finding the words*. New York: John Wiley & Sons.

Leventhal, E. A. (1996). Biology of aging. In J. Sadavoy, L. W. Lazarus, L. F. Jarvik, & G. T. Grossberg, Eds. *Comprehensive review of geriatric psychiatry–II*, (2nd ed., pp. 81–112). Washington, DC: American Psychiatric Press.

Mace, N. L., & Rabins, P. V. (1999). *The 36-hour day: a family guide to caring for persons with Alzheimer disease, related dementing illnesses and memory loss in later life* (3rd ed.). Baltimore, MD: The Johns Hopkins University Press.

Sadavoy, J., Lazarus, L. W., Jarvik, L. F., & Grossberg, G. T. (Eds.). (1996). *Comprehensive review of geriatric psychiatry–II* (2nd ed.). Washington, DC: American Psychiatric Press.

Solomon, D. H. et al. (1992). *A consumer's guide to aging*. Baltimore, MD: The Johns Hopkins University Press.

The pill book (10th ed.). (2001). New York: Bantam Books.

2000/2001 older Americans information directory (3rd ed.). (2000). Lakeville, CT: Grey House Publishing.

Weed, L. L. (1968). What physicians worry about: how to organize care of multiple problem patients. *Modern Hospital, 110*, 90–94.

CHAPTER 4

AIDS

A Fatal Virus

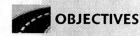

OBJECTIVES

Upon completion of this chapter, you should be able to:

- Understand the significance of AIDS, hepatitis B, and other infectious diseases for the patient and the medical system.
- Understand how caregiver anxiety may affect bystander response to EMS care.
- Explain the importance of doing a thorough assessment even when the patient is known to suffer from a chronic condition.
- Demonstrate effective listening skills.
- Explain how one's own feelings can affect professional performance.

THE CHALLENGE

The Centers for Disease Control and Prevention (CDC) estimate that there are "800,000 to 900,000 U.S. residents living with **HIV infection,** one-third of whom are unaware of their infection."[1] There are approximately 40,000 new cases of infection each year.[1] The CDC notes 23,473 cases of **AIDS** in health care workers and 453 cases in EMS providers. However, in none of the cases involving EMS providers was there documented **seroconversion** following occupational exposure.[2]

Yet, cold, impersonal statistics cannot begin to express the anguish of AIDS. Effects on patients, on communities, and on health-care workers were unprecedented in the 20th century. However, there is a precedent from the 19th century. In the 1880s and 1890s, leprosy (Hansen's disease) struck fear into the hearts of the "clean." Like AIDS patients, its victims were socially isolated and condemned. This behavior despite the fact that the disease was not highly contagious.

While AIDS is a source of concern for EMS providers, effective precautions, universally used, are effective barriers to disease transmission. These same precautions will also protect workers against the more widespread and far more communicable diseases such as **hepatitis B,** which have threatened emergency workers for decades.

The challenge of working with patients suffering from AIDS is similar, in some ways, to the challenge of working with any chronically ill patient. In other ways it is vastly different: Those newly diagnosed with AIDS tend to be young males, many under age 25. Most important, they suffer from a syndrome that baffles and terrorizes some of those on whom they must depend. The challenge is to understand and work effectively for the patient and to maintain appropriate, but not obsessive, concern for one's own safety.

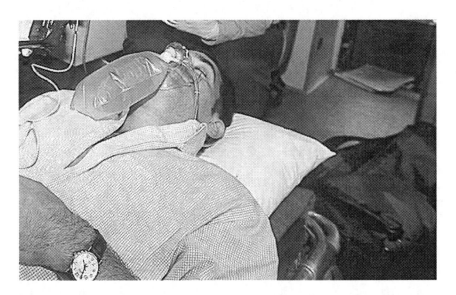

THE PATIENT AND THE SITUATION

Twenty-eight-year-old Ron Dexter lies in bed, coughing. He has a low-grade fever. In the last year he has felt his strength and his spirit wane. His will to live is gone; he finds no satisfaction in life. It seems like a decade since the clinic first told him he was HIV positive. Yet, it was only a year ago. At first he denied it. It couldn't happen to me, he thought. Yet, he knew it could. He had attended his former lover's funeral not long before he was diagnosed. Most of his heterosexual colleagues at the newspaper did not know he was gay. He wished to spare his parents the truth and to protect his "other world." He told them nothing, until his illness became so apparent that he could not hide his infirmity. Throughout his ordeal, his parents have been conspicuously absent. His sister and brother have been supportive.

He remembers his football coach's aphorism: "Life is a grindstone: it grinds you down or it polishes you up, depending on what you are made of." Old platitudes don't help him in his current situation. Life is grinding him down. His partner, John Martin, has stayed with Ron but is absorbed with his own grieving and is not fully there for him. During a recent period of remission, it appeared as if Ron might be getting the virus under control. But the recovery was short-lived. To complicate matters, Ron wonders about his responsibility for the tragedy that has engulfed them. Ron remembers his past successes and failures vividly. His memory for recent events is slipping, and he is deeply concerned about this loss.

He is not isolated, although some attention is not welcome. Friends in the AIDS Support Network have visited frequently, and their visits are encouraging. Conversely, the building superintendent seems to grow more hostile and demanding. The landlord has visited, telling Ron and John not to worry. However, he seems to be as much concerned about whether they are littering his hallways with dangerous infectious waste as he is about Ron's health.

Just as the atmosphere in the flat is melancholy today, on other days it has been thick with pain, conflict, and struggle. One reason for the melancholic atmosphere is the phone call from Dr. Moses Hallowell. Dr. Hallowell wants him to check in to Memorial Hospital, "St. Nowhere" as it is known in the gay community.

In fact, Ron is having another bout with pneumonia. He has had it before and he expects to recover—this time. However, his appetite is down, and he is sleeping way too much. His friends have remarked on his listlessness and his inability to pay attention or to remember what is happening around him. His friends attribute this to his depression. Dr. Hallowell suspects the virus is having a direct effect on Ron's brain.

John Martin is listening to soft blues in the background, as he tries to concentrate on his work. He thinks it is fortunate that he can work at home to be with Ron, but then again, he'd get more done if he were in the office. The street outside is quiet. The few children in the neighborhood are in school and most of the adults are at work. The sun shines indifferently on a mild early March day.

In sharp contrast, across town, when the Mercy ambulance dispatcher announces that Dr. Hallowell's office has called, Aerosmith is blaring from the radio in the squad room. EMS provider Mike Devereau shudders noticeably. He wishes that he, instead of his partner Lee Paulson, were driving today. Everyone at Mercy knows that Dr. Hallowell is the city's leading AIDS expert. Some EMS providers curse loudly when they receive a call to transport one of Dr. Hallowell's patients. Lee Paulson dismisses his colleagues' epithets and expletives as "just blowing off steam" before going into a tough situation. However, the anxiety that surfaces is more like lava from a volcano. It does not evaporate but leaves a covering trail destroying healthy growth.

Mike Devereau complains bitterly on the way to Clinton Street. He has a difficult time with persons with AIDS. "You know," Mike says, "my wife thinks I'm crazy doing this kind of work. I don't want a dispatch job or a desk job, but sometimes I think I should, just for her sake."

Lee sits quietly for a few seconds before answering. "Look, the last thing that a guy who's sick and dying needs is to feel that I don't want to take care of him. That just makes things worse. At least with Ron Dexter, we know what we're dealing with. It's the stabbings and shootings that frighten me. And, it's not just HIV, it's hep B and TB."

The ease with which Lee dons gloves serves to reassure Ron that, "it's not just because of my condition." As Mike readies the stretcher, Lee chats with Ron. "It must be rough, having to go back to the hospital." Ron acknowledges the fact with a half-hearted smile. Ron senses that Lee is trying to be supportive, but he feels so bad that it is difficult for him to be more involved. Lee recognizes this and is not put off. Continued conversation serves to assess Ron's degree of orientation.

John Martin remains aloof but does help with the door as they leave. Lee and Mike feel relief as they lock the stretcher into place in the ambulance. They know that they have helped a patient in need and have shown him, and themselves, what compassionate care is all about.

THE PATIENT'S WORLD

A recent public information campaign uses the stark statement "40,000,000 infected, 00,000,000 cured." This reflects the global scope of an epidemic that is considered the deadliest epidemic in human history. The bleak prospects for an AIDS patient are summarized in two words: fatal virus. Social opportunities are restricted for anyone labeled as having AIDS. This restriction extends from people diagnosed HIV positive to people with AIDS-related complex (ARC) to persons with AIDS. The disease will have economic as well as emotional effects. Even before a person can no longer work, he or she may be forced out of his or her chosen field. Once ARC or AIDS has been diagnosed, the person's subsequent behavior may reflect social isolation, economic insecurity, and anxiety associated with a deadly condition. While the possibility for psychological wellness and spiritual growth remain, the external world conspires to make them difficult to achieve. Losses tend to foster depression.

Relationships tend to be limited to a few old friends and perhaps some new friends who work in support or hospice programs. Relations with families can be problematic.

THE BEHAVIOR OF THE PATIENT

Behavior is very much related to the social and emotional situation of the patient and the progression of the illness, as well as to the patient's mental status. Disoriented patients may not care for themselves and become very disorganized. Those with depression may become suicidal; those with agitation or anger may become assaultive.

 ## THE EMOTIONS AND THOUGHTS BEHIND THE BEHAVIOR

Accommodation to AIDS often follows the pattern identified by Kübler-Ross for adaptation to other lethal illnesses: denial and isolation, anger, bargaining, depression, and acceptance.[3] Some of the characteristics of these stages are shown in Box 4–1. The EMS provider is most likely to encounter an AIDS patient during the depression stage, which is the point at which the physical ravages related to the syndrome will be most incapacitating.

It is important to consider two aspects of a patient's thinking. First, just knowing that one has AIDS, or is HIV positive, affects thinking patterns. Second, the effects of AIDS on the central nervous system may affect the patient's thinking.

BOX 4–1

STAGES IN ADAPTATION TO LETHAL ILLNESS

Frequently, a person's adaptation to lethal illness follows a five-stage process.

1. *Denial and isolation*   The patient denies the diagnosis or the prognosis and may distance himself or herself from family and friends.

2. *Anger*   The patient becomes angry at himself or herself or at others, trying to establish blame or responsibility for the illness.

3. *Bargaining*   The patient searches desperately for a cure. Often patients will make promises to God or to others about what they will do if they recover.

4. *Depression*   When the search for a cure is seen as fruitless, the patient may become depressed.

5. *Acceptance*   The final stage is often an acceptance of death as a stage of life, or even as a part of growth.

Some patients may obsess about the consequences, becoming preoccupied by thoughts of disability and death. Others may obsess about the ways in which they might have contracted AIDS and the likelihood that they have passed it on to others. There is a mental dilemma here. Patients may desperately need people but may fear betrayal. They both want and fear emotional closeness.

For some patients, guilt may be dominant. Some religious groups see AIDS as a divine judgment on an immoral lifestyle. While the AIDS patient probably does not share such a view, the questions of responsibility and guilt can loom large.

Against this background, the patient may experience symptoms of **delirium** or **dementia.** The earliest phases of dementia may show themselves as simple forgetfulness, difficulty in concentrating, or occasional problems with orientation. As neural damage progresses, the changes may become more profound. Fifty to seventy percent of AIDS patients show evidence of organic mental disorders. In extreme cases, a patient may **hallucinate,** become mute, or make up stories (confabulate), to cover memory gaps.

Ron's world is closing in on him. Physically he can do less and less. Emotionally he is depressed, he contemplates suicide, and his thoughts reveal memory and orientation deficits.

 ## FAMILY/BYSTANDER RESPONSES

Significant others will play an important role in the adaptation of a person with AIDS to his or her condition. Some will serve as patient advocates, helping the person with AIDS to negotiate the health-care system. Other persons with AIDS and their families and friends may view the health-care system suspiciously. They may see standard precautions as specific precautions and may see some routine history questions about previous illnesses as an invasion of privacy.

Some gay men are reluctant to let their parents know they have AIDS. Letting parents know might have the tragic effect of distancing them from their son at a time when he needs them. Some parents may also feel it is necessary to hide the fact that their son has AIDS.

 ## PROVIDER RESPONSES

For some EMS providers, anger, contempt, or ridicule may be the principal overt responses to persons with AIDS. However, fear of death and/or fear of spreading the disease to loved ones seem to lie behind such reactions. The physical risk of contracting AIDS is low compared to that of contracting hepatitis B. However, AIDS seems to be more feared even though hepatitis B can also be passed on to loved ones and may be fatal.

The most sensible response is preparation before the fact. While our focus is on psychological response and interaction, there are sensible physical precautions that you can take to ease doubts and eliminate sources of anxiety. First, become familiar with and use pocket masks or other shield devices during resuscitations to eliminate a major concern. Second, carry an adequate supply of vinyl or latex gloves, eye protection equipment, and a lab coat or extra jacket. Third, learn about infectious disease. Remember also that AIDS is not the only infectious disease about which you should be concerned. For hepatitis B, there is a vaccine, and vaccination is important.[4,5]

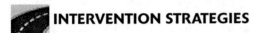 **INTERVENTION STRATEGIES**

Observe

The physical surroundings will provide clues to potential hazards and to the patient's status. Exposed needles, broken glass with blood, or other potentially infectious objects must always be treated with caution. The patient's surroundings will tell you much about the patient's likely state of mind and orientation. Well-organized living quarters suggest that the patient is continuing to adapt successfully, and may indicate continuing social support as well. Ron Dexter's living conditions seem adequate.

Interact

Sometimes prejudice against persons with AIDS leads even physicians to take inappropriate precautions. Under normal circumstances, there should be no barriers to normal interaction. AIDS is not transmitted by casual contact. EMS providers should routinely glove before any patient contact. Gloving can be done casually and appropriately, not with an exaggerated flourish. If you are comfortable in gloving with all patients, you will not give the message that this is a special precaution that you are taking because this patient is dangerous.

In fact, because of the patient's compromised immune system, he or she may have more to fear from you than you do from the patient. If you have a cold or flu and pass it on to a person with AIDS, the results can be fatal. If you are using a mask to prevent the spread of a cold, let the patients know clearly that you are doing this for their benefit.

Ask

Do not assume that an obvious chronic condition is the chief complaint. The present complaint may have little to do with the patient's compromised immune system. Relevant history will include eating and sleeping patterns, recurrent illnesses, medications, incontinence, chills, ability to move about, and current emotional state. *Questions about how a person contracted AIDS are inappropriate.*

Act

Standard precautions are always appropriate. Where possible, you should wash your hands prior to contact with the patient. Hand washing in the field can be a problem, but towelettes or foam cleaners can substitute where water is not available.

Attend

Do not stereotype. Stereotyping leads to inappropriate reactions. Operating from stereotypes of homosexuals or addicts will lead you to miss important assessment or treatment cues and will also do a disservice to your patients. One of the greatest frustrations for patients with AIDS is that they are demeaned and depersonalized in the treatment system.

Every EMS provider should develop good listening skills. Every patient, not only a person with AIDS, benefits from the opportunity to speak to a good listener. Look at the person who is speaking to you. When you are listening, your openness (or lack of it) shows through your body language and gestures. A person who is listening empathically will usually lean forward slightly; have a relaxed, rather than tense posture, and hold his or her hands open and slightly apart. Often people are forming their responses before the other person is through talking. A person who is doing this is usually tensing his body and holding his hands tightly closed together. This isn't effective listening. Box 4–2 sum-

---

BOX 4–2

SOME CHARACTERISTICS OF AN EFFECTIVE LISTENER

1. Seek to understand the person who is speaking, not simply to respond to his or her statements.

2. Listen to a person's tone and inflection as well as his or her choice of words.

3. Look at the person speaking and pay attention to body language. Does the person's body give you the same message as his or her words?

4. Don't rush in with opinions and judgments. Give the other person the freedom to express himself or herself.

5. When you speak, make it clear that you have understood what the other person has said. You can even restate the person's point more clearly than he or she might have stated it originally.

(Adapted from Covey, S. [1989]. *The seven habits of highly effective people* [pp. 235–260]. New York: Simon and Schuster.)

marizes some of the characteristics of a good listener as defined by Stephen R. Covey in *The Seven Habits of Highly Effective People.*

Document

Documentation should include all elements necessary to provide a picture of the patient's condition and your assessments and intervention activities. Document your use of standard precautions. If an unprotected exposure to blood or body fluids should occur, document the fluid to which you were exposed, the route of exposure, and any actions you took to reduce the risk. If you are exposed to contaminated body fluids, your exposure should be reported to the designated safety officer in your agency. Precautionary treatment should be sought and documented appropriately. You should know your agency's policies for reporting an occupational exposure. Blood contact with intact skin is not a danger. Only when there is dermatitis, a cut, or some other loss of skin integrity would there be a potential danger of infection.

 CONSIDERATIONS FOR EMS PROVIDERS

Negative emotional reactions to persons with AIDS are unhelpful to patients and to EMS providers. Such reactions lead to inferior, inadequate care and to burnout. Emergency work brings you face to face with people under stress. Some of them are under greater stress than you can possibly imagine. Judging the person on the basis of nondisease characteristics is a sure route to treatment care failure.

Nagging doubts and the negative feelings are real. Ignoring them is also a route to treatment failure. There are concerns about contracting and spreading infectious disease. Emergency care will be stronger when we confront these concerns and resolve them. The best way to do this is through education. AIDS is not only a challenge to us as health-care workers and to the health-care system, it is also a challenge to society as a whole.

CONCLUSION

It may seem hard to believe that in the mid-1980s, people were asking if fear of AIDS would destroy emergency-care systems as we knew them. Responders rose above the pessimism of those days to the point where standard precautions are second nature. Today's EMS providers and their patients are better protected and better served.

REVIEW QUESTIONS

1. What are the typical stages in adaptation to a fatal illness?
2. How might knowing that a person is HIV positive affect his or her family?
3. When EMS providers (or others) joke about AIDS, what might this indicate?
4. In what ways, if any, should an EMS provider treat a person with HIV differently than other patients?
5. List at least three important characteristics of effective listening.

EXERCISES

1. Have a group discussion on the pros and cons of a needle exchange program.
2. Have an HIV/AIDS patient address your group. You will hear some powerful and amazing stories.
3. Visit a neonatal unit where there are HIV positive babies. A very moving experience.

REFERENCES

1. National Institute of Allergy and Infectious Disease, National Institute of Health (May 2001) Fact Sheet, HIV infection and AIDS: an overview. Office of Communications and Public Liaison. www.niaid.nih.gov/factsheets/hivinfo.htm.
2. Centers for Disease Control and Prevention (2001). Surveillance of health care workers with HIV/AIDS. National Center for HIV, STD, and TB Prevention. www.cdc.gov/hiv/pubs/facts/hcwsurv.htm.
3. Kübler-Ross, E. (1997). *AIDS: the ultimate challenge.* New York: Macmillan.
4. Bixler, D., Butwin, J., Mallatt, M., Naylor, D., Quintana, C., Shoemaker, S., & Steele, G. (2002).*Infectious Disease Exposure Manual for Emergency Response Employees.* www.in.gov/isdh/publications/pubs/emermanu.htm.
5. Nixon, R. G. (2000). *Communicable diseases and infection control.* Upper Saddle River, NJ: Prentice Hall.

FURTHER INFORMATION

Internet Resources

Centers for Disease Control and Prevention: www.cdc.gov

HIV/AIDS information: www.thebody.com

Massachusetts Department of Public Health: www.state.ma.us/dph/dphhome.htm

Media Resources

Movies

And the Band Played On

Philadelphia

Longtime Companion

Books

Broder, S. & Merigan, T. C., Jr. (1994). *Textbook of AIDS medicine* (12th ed.). Baltimore: Lippincott Williams and Wilkins.

Garrett, L. (1999). *Coming plague: newly emerging diseases in a world out of balance*. New York: Viking Penguin.

Stine, G. J. (2001). *AIDS update*. Englewood Cliffs, NJ: Prentice Hall.

CHAPTER 5

Trauma

More Than Physical Injury

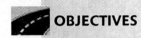 **OBJECTIVES**

Upon completion of this chapter, you should be able to:

- Understand the significance of trauma in society and in your work.
- Explain how a patient's subjective response to injury may be quite different from that of the emergency-care team.
- Explain the importance of considering preexisting medical conditions in the assessment process.
- Demonstrate effective communication while considering the physical needs of the patient.

THE CHALLENGE

In the United States, more than 100,000 people die of injuries each year. This statistic makes injury the leading cause of death for persons between the ages of 1 and 44. However, fatalities are just the tip of the iceberg. Each year millions of persons will need medical attention for an injury.[1]

A trauma patient presents many challenges to an EMS provider. The first challenge may be reaching the patient safely. Darkness, poor weather, and environmental hazards, such as downed power lines and tight spaces, complicate your task. The second challenge may be completing a systematic assessment and beginning necessary care, including spinal immobilization, in such an environment. Third, patients often behave unpredictably. This behavior may be due to the nature of the injury or to alcohol or other drug intoxication at the time of injury.[2] It may also arise from anxiety following the injury when a patient realizes the possible consequences of the injury including disfigurement, loss of independence, or financial difficulty.[3] You must respond realistically to these concerns while providing prompt emergency care for injuries suffered.

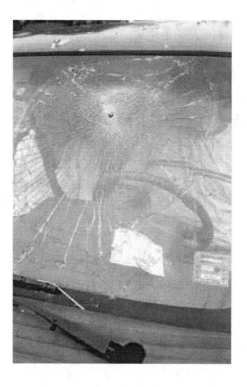

 ## THE PATIENT AND THE SITUATION

Shortly after 11:00 P.M. on Saturday night, Paul Butterworth, age 23, is heading down Route 110. A light rain is falling. He is slightly over the speed limit of 45 miles per hour. He would be driving faster, but he is trying to prove to his fiancee, Dawn Hurst, how responsible he is. Dawn has been ignoring him since they quarreled earlier over his drinking. Alcohol is a serious complication in their relationship. Paul sees nothing wrong with "a couple of beers" at a party, while Dawn is sensitive to any drinking. Her father was a binge drinker who would go off on drinking sprees and wreak havoc on the family. Dawn confronted Paul early in the evening about having too much to drink. He had four beers in 2 hours. Dawn knew that if Paul continued drinking at that rate, he would be over the limit by the time they left the party. They left shortly after this confrontation.

Dawn is thinking about ice skating on Sunday. Paul is sulking. Both are angry. Paul moves the Olds through the S curves down Mile Hill. A small animal darts out in front of them. He swerves, then brakes, but it is too late. The car crashes into the stone retaining wall. Paul's chest strikes the steering wheel, and, still propelled forward, his head hits the windshield. He was not wearing a seat belt. Dawn, who was wearing her seat belt, has wrenched her wrist and twisted her right foot as she braced herself for the impact.

Mabel Humphries lives nearby. She hears the crash and immediately calls the sheriff's office. She knows the number well. She has called Sheriff Tucker before. Mabel dresses rapidly and runs across the road. She reaches Paul's car just as Paul and Dawn start to stir. "You alright in there?" she calls. Dawn answers, "I'm OK." Paul responds more slowly, and Mabel cannot understand what he said. She thinks he is drunk and doesn't press it. "You youngsters just sit there; help is on the way."

Paul and Dawn sit in silence. The anger has gone, but the silence borne of disbelief and injury is as oppressive.

Across town, Willow Creek's two on-call volunteer EMS providers are dressing. Helen Johnson has been in bed since 10 o'clock. The call broke into her dream sleep. She is groggy, but comes around quickly. Steve Goodnow, the other volunteer on call was still up, catching the end of the late movie. Steve generally stays up until 1:30 A.M. or so on the weekend nights when he's on duty. Often he misses the end of the late show.

Steve and Helen head out to "The S's." As they exchange pleasantries, Steve learns of Helen's annoyance. She always feels uncomfortable on runs like this. "I hope it's not one of those kids, tanked up and speeding." Steve is about to say, "It goes with the territory," but he does not. He knows that 2 years ago, Helen worked a fatal accident on Route 13. A 17-year-old girl was killed. Her boyfriend, an 18-year-old, was uninjured but was so drunk he could barely stand. He faced only charges of drinking while intoxicated (DWI) and not vehicular homicide charges. Steve ducks the subject.

Paul Butterworth tries to move but falls back into the seat. He tries to explain that he had to swerve, but his explanation makes no sense to Dawn or to Mabel. Dawn is now fully alert and is concerned about the sharp, persistent pain in her right ankle.

Dawn has strangely conflicted feelings. She is furious at Paul, but she is also concerned about his potentially serious injury. She is furious at herself for not insisting even earlier than Paul switch to soft drinks. She is concerned that she has suffered a crippling and possibly disabling injury herself. The idea of the skating competition on Sunday flashes through her mind.

Paul gathers his strength and forces his weight against the door. It yields. He steps onto the road just as a police cruiser arrives. Officer Horning places his cruiser behind Paul's car as a warning to other traffic. He helps Paul to the side of the road. The ambulance arrives almost simultaneously with the police.

Paul attempts to get up. The policeman places him on his back, suggesting he might injure himself further if he moves around. "What about Dawn?" Paul asks. Horning suddenly remembers there might be more victims. As Helen and Steve approach, the officer says he hasn't had time to check the car; there may be someone else inside. Helen figures that Paul is the driver. She can see a woman sitting nearly upright in the front passenger seat. She tells Dawn to remain still when she opens the door. There is no one else in the car, and no sign that there were passengers in the back seat. She introduces herself, tells Dawn that her partner is helping a man by the side of the road, and asks if there was anyone else involved in the crash. Dawn says, "No."

"My ankle. I broke something, I'm sure." Helen tells her to keep still. After properly immobilizing Dawn's head and neck, she will examine her for any injuries and treat what she finds. She explains that she wants to treat Dawn's ankle but first has to check to make sure there are no other injuries. The rapid trauma assessment is unremarkable except for a pain in the wrist and ankle tenderness. She splints Dawn's wrist and ankle rapidly and goes to join Steve. On nights like this she wishes more volunteers would show up.

Steve and the officer are placing Paul on a long spineboard. Paul's immobilization is complicated by his disorientation and changes in mood. Nevertheless, Steve continues to talk to him and to ask him questions. At times Paul cannot remember what time it is or even where he is. When Paul is immobilized, Helen and Steve lift the board to the ambulance cot, secure it, and transfer Paul to the ambulance.

Helen sees that Mabel Humphries is worried. Before they leave, she reassures Mabel that they are doing all they can for the two young victims. Helen assures Mabel that she did the right thing. Now they will go to Carpenterville where the emergency department (ED) will determine what else Paul and Dawn require.

Postscript

Paul, because of his head injury, faces an uncertain course of treatment. He suffered a subdural hematoma, requiring surgical intervention. The head injury was serious enough that he experiences mood swings and memory problems even several months later. Dawn will skate again but not this season. She will have new concerns about parties and drinking. At the hospital Paul's blood alcohol level was 0.05. He was not legally intoxicated, but for Dawn, the accident has further confirmed the dangers of alcohol. She broke off her relationship with Paul one month after the accident.

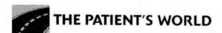 **THE PATIENT'S WORLD**

Unintentional injuries occur, by definition, when they are not expected, which does not mean that injuries cannot be prevented through safety engineering or public education.[4] However, it does mean that they interrupt and transform the patient's world. Generally, an injured person was engaged in some typical, familiar activity such as driving, walking, playing a sport, or working prior to the injury. The crash brought Paul and Dawn into a world far different from the one they inhabited just moments before. The precrash behaviors—making a point with an accusatory silence; defending one's behavior—are now irrelevant. A new set of behaviors, thoughts, and emotions are now important.

 ## THE BEHAVIOR OF THE PATIENT

Immediately following a crash or injury, the first reaction is often absence of movement, a numbness. As the initial numbness wears off, each injured person, based on preinjury activities and the nature of individual injuries, responds differently.

For Paul, his incongruous reactions, including incoherence and the attempt to flee, are related to his head injury. His earlier drinking and his emotional fight with Dawn complicate the picture. The behavior of a head-injured patient is directly influenced by the injury. Massive trauma will result in coma; less severe trauma will result in momentary unconsciousness followed by swings in activity levels. Some head-injured patients become belligerent, combative, and hostile. Their inability to comprehend what is happening can bring forth a violent response. Others may withdraw and attempt to isolate themselves. Others may actively attempt to flee the scene. It is essential to recognize that behavior can fluctuate and that the submissive patient may become wildly agitated without any apparent aggravation.

Dawn focuses on her swollen, possibly fractured ankle. She worries about Paul and herself; yet she is also angry with him and wants nothing to do with him. In cases of extremity trauma, the pain of the obvious injury dominates patients' reactions. They may protect the injured limb and expect immediate relief of the obvious injury. Frequently they resent any attempt to assess or treat other injuries. Some patients, however, may be reluctant even to look at the source of their pain.

 ## THE EMOTIONS AND THOUGHTS BEHIND THE BEHAVIOR

Some emotional traits are related to accident-proneness. **Impulsivity,** aggressiveness, low frustration tolerance, self-centeredness, and recklessness may lead individuals to become involved in situations in which injuries are likely.

The absence of movement immediately after an accident is associated with disbelief that an accident has occurred and absence of emotion. The mind attempts to handle overwhelming stress by an emotional shock mechanism. The psyche is pushed too far by the devastation and the pain, responding with a numbness that provides temporary relief. To an outsider this patient's affect may seem seriously inappropriate. It is important to recognize that each victim–patient begins to come to grips with the consequences in his or her own time. Just when the emotional shock will wear off cannot be predicted. Many patients will have passed through this phase by the time rescue workers appear on scene.

Following the period of psychic numbing, individual personality factors and history determine the reaction. Dawn handles her stress in a characteristic way. She anticipates the worst and becomes obsessed by this possibility. Dawn believes she will never skate again.

The emotional response of the head-injured patient is, as the description of behavior suggests, erratic. Emotions will vary even from moment to moment. One moment the patient may feel like crying (and do so); the next, the patient may be gripped by an uncontrollable desire to laugh.

Head trauma affects orientation and recall. The more severe the head trauma, the greater the disorientation. Knowledge of date and time are first to go, followed by knowledge of place. Knowledge of name is the last to go. At certain moments, Paul did not know what the date was or where he was. The more severe the trauma, the greater the memory loss. Immediate recall is first to go, then recent memory, then long-term memory. If the patient has been involved with alcohol or other drugs, the thought disturbances are compounded, making assessment even more difficult.

Although pain is a critical factor in the emotional response, anger and grief may also be important. A patient may mourn the loss of ability to function. He or she may grieve over a "dead" limb and feel that nothing will ever be right again. For Dawn, the potential loss of her ability to skate is a cause to grieve. She fears important future possibilities are dead. Other patients may be ashamed of their injuries. A patient may feel ashamed that his or her clothes have been cut away by strangers or that he or she needs help getting into the ambulance.

Patients often relive the moments before the incident. As they explore these moments, they often find fault with themselves or with someone else. Dawn blames Paul. She also blames herself for not making him leave the party earlier. Then she wonders if she has been too hard on him: was their argument really responsible for the accident? These guilty thoughts complicate psychological and physical recovery for many. In some cases, these thoughts may become obsessive for the victim. The pattern becomes, "If I hadn't done this, then this wouldn't have happened." Later, they may experience flashbacks. This tendency to relive the incident may also show up in painful nightmares later.

Finally, those who live through an accident in which others have died may experience survivor guilt. It is often difficult for a patient to admit such a feeling let alone to talk about it.

FAMILY/BYSTANDER RESPONSES

Families and friends experience the full gamut of emotions. Many experience greater anxiety than the physically injured victims. The uninjured person, not feeling the pain of the injury, may fantasize about the seriousness of the trauma and let his or her imagination run wild in the absence of physical information. As with many other emergency situations, the family may feel responsible, and guilty. They may find themselves obsessed with the incident. They may also experience flashbacks to the time when they first heard about the event and relive the scene in all its horror.

To complete the picture, it is important to consider bystanders. Most accidents attract bystanders. Even bystanders can be psychologically traumatized by the event. Many of us became deeply, physically affected by the scene of Ground Zero, the site of the World Trade Center catastrophe. One does not need to be physically injured to be hurt.

As every EMS provider knows, bystanders will show a range of behaviors from the helpful to the distracting to the downright obstructive. Some rush forward to offer help. Perhaps the best help they can give is to go elsewhere to seek more competent help. They may complicate the patient's condition by improper movement. Other bystanders may wander aimlessly about, overwhelmed by the event. Still others look for guidance. They desire to help but feel incompetent to intervene.

 PROVIDER RESPONSES

Accidents do happen. Prevention-oriented practitioners are right to emphasize risk factors, and epidemiologists can identify conditions that make trauma more likely, but psychologically, once the accident has occurred, it does not help the patients or the helpers to assign blame. It does help to understand contributing factors that can also contribute to the way in which the patient presents to you.

There are three lessons to take into—and away from—a serious injury scene. First, it is all too possible to lose sight of the patient as a person. Of course, injuries must be assessed and treated, but successful treatment requires honest interaction as well as prompt action.

Second, your emotional state or prejudices based on past experience prior to the incident can, if not recognized, affect your response to the patients. In our story, Helen went into the scene somewhat angry about being on duty. Her stresses could have carried over to her relationship with her partner and her treatment of Dawn. An EMS provider who dislikes people who don't seatbelt their children cannot let this affect intervention.

Finally, EMS providers, like family and bystanders, are affected by what they see and feel at an accident scene. They may also experience flashbacks and moments of self-doubt. Helen and Steve might recall the incident every time they drive through the S curves.

 ## INTERVENTION STRATEGIES

Observe

It is essential to size up the scene as well as assess the obvious patients. If you are first on the scene, where you place your ambulance is important. Watch for hazards such as electrical wires, leaking gasoline, potentially dangerous traffic conditions, or for signs that the accident might have been caused by hazards in the road. It is also essential to look for any victims who have been thrown from or have wandered away from the scene of the accident. Finally, don't overlook the back set. Check for children who may have been thrown to the floor or who may be hiding.

Interact

As the situation permits, begin with a formal introduction. Remember that the patient's confidence may be fostered as much through interaction as by your technical skills. Remember also that the ambulance, the lights, the radios, and even the presence of uniformed personnel can be intimidating. Explain what you are doing and why, as far as possible. Keeping up a conversation and monitoring for level of pain not only involves the patient in care but gives you important information about the patient's level of consciousness and airway status.

Ask

Even if the cause of the accident seems obvious, ask the patient what happened. The reason why the driver lost control of the car may not be obvious. Ask about mechanisms of injury. Patients may experience whiplash or **coup-contrecoup** injuries. An obvious injury on the right side of the head may have been preceded by a violent thrust to the left with rebound to the right. Further, do not assume that an obvious injury is the only one or even the most important one. Consider the possibility of internal injuries.

There is also a second reason for asking about the crash situation. It can be a natural second step in assessing the patient's level of consciousness. First, ask for the patient's name when you introduce yourself. Second, determine if the patient knows where he or she is and what has happened. Third, see if the patient can tell you the day, date, and time.

Get a medical history. Medications that alter perception, illnesses that affect coordination, and drugs that impair judgment are important factors in accidents. They also affect the way the patient will appear to you. Sleeping pills, antihistamines, barbiturates, tranquilizers, steroids, and other medications can produce similar disorientation. Other medical conditions that can produce disorientation include seizure disorders, strokes, central nervous system infections, tumors, and blood sugar imbalances. Obviously, alcohol, cocaine, phencyclidine (PCP), hallucinogens, and opiates alter consciousness. Knowledge of other medical conditions such as epilepsy, heart disease, other recent trauma or surgery, neurologic disorders, allergies, and current medications is important. Asking about pregnancy, if it is a possibility, is also important.

Act

Whatever the patient's condition, it is important to take appropriate infection control precautions. If there are broken glass or twisted metal hazards, it may be important to use heavy-duty gloves in addition to latex or vinyl gloves and any simple protective clothing necessary.

Attend

As well as listening to what the patient says in answer to your questions, it is important to listen to the questions that the patient asks or the statements that he or she makes. You cannot tell Dawn if she will ever skate again; however, you can recognize that this is an important, emotional issue for Dawn and answer her on that level. You cannot tell Mabel Humphries that the victims will be all right, but you can recognize Mabel's real concern that she did everything she could do. Where citizens have helped—perhaps by calling for help appropriately—you can confirm this and let them know they are appreciated.

Document

It is important to document suspected mechanisms of injury for two reasons. First, the more an ED physician or a surgeon knows about the crash conditions and mechanism of injury, the better he or she can assess and treat less obvious injuries. Second, more hospitals are using special codes called E codes in epidemiologic studies. These studies are valuable in developing injury prevention programs. Much of the information required can be reported by EMS providers. Furthermore, taking vital signs, calculating trauma scores, and doing mental status examinations at several times during transport will help to assess whether the patient is deteriorating. As in the cardiac run, run times are linked to survival, especially time from call to definitive care.

 CONSIDERATIONS FOR EMS PROVIDERS

Trauma calls can leave emotional scars on the helpers as well as the victims. This is recognized in critical incident stress debriefing (CISD), and many progressive departments include valuable debriefing procedures for following up emotionally wrenching runs. However, garden-variety trauma takes its toll. A good rescuer, confronted by too many drunk drivers, may become hardened and cynical. A series of calls to the same intersection can trigger flashbacks or unwanted memories when passing the dangerous spot.

The first line of treatment is recognition. Recognize that exposure to pain and suffering takes a toll. EMS providers can react inappropriately to persons in pain in a number of ways. These are summarized in Box 5–1. Holding in the emotional pain allows it to form the equivalent of an infection. Instead of poisoning the blood, it poisons attitudes and relationships.

Regular review sessions may be one of the most effective ways to address the emotional response to trauma and to keep EMS providers current in trauma care. Critiques that focus constructively on all aspects of EMS intervention from observation to documentation will not only improve trauma patient care but will also contribute to your professional growth.

Finally, know when to call for more help. One of the greatest stressors is to find oneself with too many patients and too few resources. Policies and procedures should spell out the conditions under which it is appropriate to call for a second unit or for mutual aid backup. There is another sense in which it is important to know when to call for more help. This is when an EMS provider's problems are more difficult than the resources that the service can muster to deal with them. Here, outside assistance from knowledgeable clergy, psychologists, or psychiatrists may be necessary.

BOX 5–1

INAPPROPRIATE RESPONSES TO PERSONS IN PAIN

Abstraction	Focusing on surrounding conditions rather than listening to the person in pain
Pity	Thinking about the person's characteristics that make him or her different from us: "The poor unfortunates"
Professional warmth	Responding with "impersonal friendliness" (a studied set of emotional responses that do not really consider the individual patient)
Compulsive hyperactivity	Keeping so busy that there is no time to attend to the person in pain

(Adapted from Dass, R. & Gorman, P. [1991]. How can I help? New York: Alfred A Knopf, p. 64.)

CONCLUSION

So much attention has been focused on multiple system trauma and systems of trauma care that it is easy to forget that most injuries will not require the services of an advanced life-support team and a fully mobilized system. However, injuries that look trivial to a seasoned emergency medical professional can seem devastating to the patient.

REVIEW QUESTIONS

1. How might injury affect a person's self-image?
2. How might injury change relationships between the injured person and significant others?
3. What are some of the inappropriate responses an EMS provider might make to a person in pain?
4. What are some of the consequences of poor documentation in trauma care?

EXERCISES

1. Have a survivor of a major trauma address your group. Stories of courage and persevering.
2. Visit an orthopedic ward.
3. Visit a rehabilitation hospital. Stories of courage and not giving up.
4. Under what circumstances might an EMS provider blame the patient for his or her injuries?

REFERENCES

1. National Institute of General Medical Sciences Fact Sheet, www.nigms.nih.gov/news.
2. Avis, H. (1999). *Drugs and life,* (4th ed.). Boston: WCB McGraw-Hill.
3. Hubble, M. W., & Hubble, J. D. (2001). *Principles of advanced trauma care.* Clifton Park, NY: Delmar Learning.

FURTHER INFORMATION

Internet Resources

American College of Surgeons: www.facs.org

American College of Emergency Physicians: www.acep.org

Media Resources

Movies

Born on the Fourth of July

The Water Dance

The Other Side of the Mountain

Television Series

Trauma: Life in the ER on The Learning Channel

Third Watch a television series on NBC

Books

Nutt, D., Davidson, J. R. T., & Zohar, J. (Eds.). (2000). *Post-traumatic stress disorder: diagnosis, management and treatment.* Boston: Blackwell Science.

Wilson, J. P., Friedmen, U. J., & Lindy, J. D. (Eds.). (2001). *Treating psychological trauma and PTSD.* New York: Guilford Press.

CHAPTER 6

Rape

Hidden Injuries

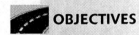

OBJECTIVES

Upon completion of this chapter, you should be able to:

- Understand why the rates of reported rape may be much lower than the actual incidence of rape.
- Understand the emotional as well as the physical consequences of rape.
- Demonstrate effective, but respectful, collection of important patient information.
- Explain the importance of documentation.

THE CHALLENGE

In 2000, 261,000 people were the victims of rape, attempted rape, or sexual assault. Of that 261,000, 114,000 were victims of sexual assault, 55,000 were victims of attempted rape, and 92,000 were victims of rape.[1] However, there is strong evidence that most rapes are not reported.

The psychological pain of intentionally inflicted trauma is often more far-reaching than that which results from an accident. When you respond to a rape or sexual assault, you have a great opportunity to address both the physical and the psychological pain. Yet you face special challenges in emergency medical care of a sexually assaulted patient. These include:

- Gaining the patient's trust
- Performing an assessment on a patient who is sensitive to any perceived violation of privacy

- Effectively supporting the patient during treatment
- Dealing with your own feelings

You can have a tremendous influence on the patient's decisions and, therefore, on the patient's ultimate recovery from the emotional trauma of assault.

In the following pages we present a vignette concerning rape. You can apply many of the patient responses, assessment, and care concepts we describe here to a wide variety of situations involving intentional injury, including victims of assault, survivors of hostage situations, and people who have been tortured.

THE PATIENT AND THE SITUATION

Jennifer Collins is lying against the wall in the lobby of her Victorian-style apartment house. She is sobbing. Her clothes are in disarray. It is 10:55 P.M., Thursday, September 28. Her life changed dramatically when she returned to her apartment building 15 minutes ago.

After attending an evening college course, she enjoyed a cup of coffee with friends and returned home later than usual. As she entered the vestibule of her building, she was suddenly set on by a man entering behind her. She told herself, "It can't be happening to me!" At first, she thought it was a prank. As the shadowy figure continued to force himself on her, she realized it was no prank. Initially she parried his movements and hit him with her bag. She gasped—

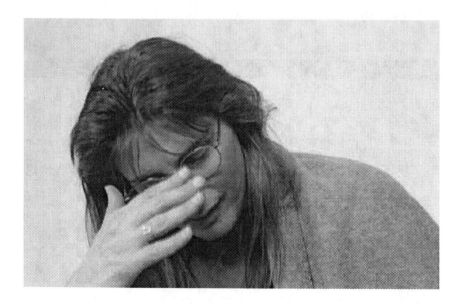

weakly, nervously—then her mind went blank. She felt as if she would pass out; her cry for help was almost inaudible. She wanted to run away but could not.

She vividly relives the moment when it "got serious." He grabbed her left arm firmly, turned her to face him, shook her, and slammed her body against the door to the basement.

She hoped that it was just a mugging. She knew she could survive a robbery—if he would just stop hurting her. Now Jennifer wavers between amnesia and vivid recollection of the events of the last half hour. "The knife! The knife!" she shouts aloud. For one brief moment she relives her attacker's death threat, although she has no clear idea where the knife came from. She can recall nothing after the sight of the knife except his rough treatment of her and his threat, "If you try anything, you little bitch, you're dead meat!"

As she lies in the hallway, she is afraid, ashamed, and haunted by the fear that the attacker will come back.

Jennifer is **ambivalent** about what she wants now: She wants to go to her apartment; but she doesn't want to be alone. She wants her mother, but she never wants her mother to know what happened to her. She wants her boyfriend Frank to tell her everything is all right, but she doesn't want any man to touch her.

Finally, she staggers to the second-floor landing and knocks on the door. No one answers, but she knows that the Allens are in. They watch the late show in bed every night. She cries, she screams, she sits in front of the door. Mrs. Allen calls out from behind the door, "Who's there?" "It's me, Jennie. From upstairs. I've been ra. . . ." She cannot utter that word.

Once in the apartment she wails and paces. Mrs. Allen quickly calls the police emergency number. A police car arrives within 2 minutes. Jennie sees the officers as a threat rather than as allies. The officers are courteous and professional, but they cannot get any information from Jennie.

The third service EMS was alerted directly by the police dispatcher. The EMS providers arrive within a minute of the police. Betty James and Henry Williams have only worked together twice before, but each has a good sense of the other's strengths and weaknesses. Betty has already decided she will take the lead here. Betty has volunteered with the rape crisis team at the hospital. She has seen other women who have experienced the trauma that Jennie is now going through. The police officers also know of Betty's work and trust her to handle this situation appropriately. She wants to be there for Jennifer. Henry Williams grew up in a small rural community where rape was never discussed, and except for "bad girls," sexual intimacy followed marriage. Henry is uncomfortable in this situation. He knows that Ms. Collins needs their help and is glad to have Betty James along on this call.

Betty introduces herself and Henry. At first, Jennie further withdraws, then she embraces Betty as if she were her only friend in the world. "Help me," she sobs. "Keep those men away. Don't let them see me like this."

As Jennie holds on to Betty, the whole incident suddenly passes before her eyes. The vivid reliving is over in a flash; then she feels blank. "I want my mother. I want to see Frank."

Jennifer eagerly embraced Betty when she first came in. Just as suddenly, she abruptly detaches herself and exclaims. "What are you doing here?" She adjusts her blouse and skirt and acts as if nothing has happened. There is a tense silence as everyone reorganizes their thoughts and reactions. Henry thinks that Jennifer is hysterical. Betty understands this is a common reaction. Betty cautiously responds. "You must be hurting. We are emergency medical providers. We want to help. Can we help you?" Jennifer responds with tears, thinking. "This is so unreal."

The police officer has been standing in the background. Seeing Jennifer's acquiescence, he interrupts. "If you can tell us something about the man who attacked you, we can alert the other units to look out for him. Then we'll go to the hospital." Jennifer senses Betty's concern and also senses that the police officer is impatient. She is caught between wanting help and wanting to be left alone.

Betty suggests that Mrs. Allen put on some coffee and that she and Jennifer just sit quietly for a few minutes. Jennie pleads, "What do I do now?" Betty catches herself just as she is about to outline the rest of her planned intervention. "What do you mean?" she asks. Jennifer realizes she has some control. By allowing Jennifer to know she has—and will continue to have—a say in the process, Betty is confirming her independence.

Jennie responds, "Do I go to the hospital? Do I talk to the police? My boyfriend will kill me if he finds out I was out this late all alone." Betty shares her experiences at the rape crisis center. She describes the advantages of an assessment here and a thorough assessment at the emergency department (ED). She reminds Jennifer that she will be with her all the way to the hospital, if Jennifer wants to go there. Betty describes what the ED will do. She notes that Jennifer is not paying attention. Jennifer says, "What about my boyfriend?" Then she is silent. Her selective inattention suggests to Betty that she has already decided to go to the ED. Her mind is racing ahead, thinking of the further consequences of going for treatment. Her boyfriend is still a problem for her. Betty confirms that Jennifer wants to go to the hospital. Jennifer makes another decision. She tells the officer—to his great relief—that she will give him a full report at the hospital.

"What about Frank?" Jennifer asks. Betty replies, "What do you want to do?" In a moment of courage and hope, she announces that she wants him to know. Betty suggests that a counselor at the hospital can help her with this.

Betty conducts a thorough but sensitive examination. She discovers that Jennifer has bruises on her back and arms and complains of pain in her thighs. Her vital signs are within normal limits. Betty explains that it is company policy that all patients must be carried down stairs in a stair chair. Jennie agrees.

Jennifer rides in a semisitting position. Betty holds her hand all the way to the hospital.

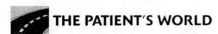

 THE PATIENT'S WORLD

Until 40 minutes ago, Jennie Collins lived in much the same world as any other career woman in her midtwenties with an interest in continuing her education and a serious romantic involvement. Nothing Jennie did invited an attack. Nothing has prepared her for this shattering experience and the work that will be involved in repairing her life. Reported rapes have increased dramatically, but many attacks still go unreported (see Box 6–1).

THE BEHAVIOR OF THE PATIENT

Although it has only been 40 minutes since the attack began, to Jennie it seems like a year since she last felt right. She traveled through a foyer and up a flight of stairs, but she feels as if she has climbed a mountain. The very real threat of death—the confrontation with eternity—changed all.

On the one hand, a victim of rape frequently wants to run and hide, to be invisible, but she also wants someone to comfort her. To flee or to accept comfort is the dilemma for the victim of a sexual assault. Flight can take many forms. It may involve actually running from the scene; it may involve partial amnesia for the event. It may mean a chemical retreat through alcohol or tranquilizers. On the other hand, the victim may seek support and security from someone who will not hurt her. She is often unsure as to whom she needs— mother, friend, lover, concerned stranger. In this context, she can be encouraged to turn to competent professionals such as a rape crisis center and family. You can be instrumental in getting the victim to accept treatment and in setting the stage for later recovery.[2] Box 6–2 summarizes the reasons that a rape victim should seek medical treatment.

BOX 6–1

FOUR REASONS WHY A VICTIM MAY NOT WANT TO REPORT A RAPE

1. It may be difficult for her to talk about the experience to the police.
2. Repeating the story may cause her to relieve the assault experience.
3. The rapist might be an acquaintance or even a husband or ex-husband.
4. The victim might be an undocumented resident.

THREE REASONS WHY A RAPE VICTIM SHOULD SEEK MEDICAL TREATMENT

1. It is necessary to determine if the victim has been physically injured.

2. It is necessary to ease fears, such as fears about venereal disease, unwanted pregnancy, or AIDS, and to take appropriate measures.

3. It is essential to collect medical evidence to prosecute the rapist if and when a suspect is caught.

 ## THE EMOTIONS AND THOUGHTS BEHIND THE BEHAVIOR

Perhaps the victim's greatest fear is that there is no resolution for the fear and the pain: the fear that neither flight nor comfort offer any real hope. In other words, the fear that she is powerless.

Unless the victim works through the event successfully, either alternative may have unhealthy consequences. The dangers of flight responses have been noted previously. Comfort seeking may lead to an inability to tolerate being alone, to excessive dependence on others, and to a need to be perpetually busy.

The thoughts and feelings that follow an assault and plague the victim for months after may be debilitating. The immediate thoughts and feelings may include emotional shock (numbness), disbelief, embarrassment, shame, guilt, depression, and disorientation, as well as powerlessness.[3,4] These reactions are shown in Box 6–3. Denial, flashbacks, intrusive thoughts, fears of another assault, and nightmares may persist. Seemingly small cues can trigger mighty responses.

The victim may blame herself or others as she searches for explanations. Jennie may come to believe that something she did, said, or forgot to do provoked or exacerbated the attack. The victim can become a victim of her own self-examination. Closely related to this phenomenon is the tendency to blame others—to find external causes: a neighbor who should have come to her aid; a landlord who should have provided better security; the police for failing to patrol the neighborhood more carefully. A person who is overwhelmed will often seek out someone else to blame. In a drastic extension of blame, Jennie may see all men or even society as the cause of her victimization. Such reactions may make physical and emotional intimacy difficult.

A victim may have some very practical fears as well. She may have very real concerns about pregnancy or sexually transmitted diseases or AIDS.

BOX 6–3

IMMEDIATE EMOTIONAL REACTIONS TO SEXUAL ASSAULT

Powerlessness	Shame
Emotional shock (numbness)	Guilt
Disbelief	Depression
Embarrassment	Disorientation

It is important to recognize that rape is a crime of violence, not of passion.[3] It is usually violence toward a woman by a man with the objectives of dominating, inflicting pain, and humiliating her, not reaching orgasm. Assailants often plan the act in advance. Their selection of a victim may have more to do with the situation than the victim's characteristics: Some victims are girls under twelve; others are elderly.

Given the violent, potentially homicidal context, you must remember that whatever steps a victim took to save her life were all right. It is important that the victim appreciate that survival is the paramount concern. Yet many survivors become critical of their behavior and the measures they took to save their lives.

 ## FAMILY/BYSTANDER RESPONSES

The assault victim may have several conflicting feelings about her responsibility for what has occurred, and she will be very sensitive to the responses of her family and loved ones and even unrelated bystanders.

Family members, friends, and lovers may respond to the rape victim (or the victim of any physical assault) in one of three very different ways. One response is to blame the victim, for instance, to accuse her of not taking the proper precautions to prevent the attack. Such accusations can be brutally direct: "You should have known better than to. . . . !" or relatively subtle: "If only you had. . . ."

Another response is to withdraw, to become aloof and emotionally distant. When family members of friends seem to be withdrawing, it may be because they have trouble dealing with another's pain. One person might deal with this discomfort by busying himself or herself with some task that does not require close contact with the victim. Such behavior can affect the victim negatively; she may misinterpret the withdrawal as disapproval.

The third response, active support, is much more desirable. Active support involves listening, responding to the victim's expressed needs and concerns, and letting the victim make her own decisions, as far as that is possible.

 PROVIDER RESPONSES

EMS providers, like families, friends, and coworkers, typically respond in one of three ways: supportive, aloof, or accusatory. Support is a welcome response, bolstering a damaged sense of self and promoting recovery. The supportive EMS providers listen, they are willing to spend time, and they will open their hearts when the victim pours her heart out. An aloof response generally involves ignoring or minimizing the situation, and focusing on the physical injury rather than the mental or spiritual ones. Accusatory responses suggest that the victim invited the attack by going where she shouldn't have gone or by dressing or behaving provocatively. The victim can become the victim of her helpers or loved ones.

 INTERVENTION STRATEGIES

Observe

The scene can yield important patient care information. In a violent attack, the victim may have suffered injuries from being thrown or pushed against walls, doors, or radiators. You should suspect blunt injuries as well as direct injuries from hitting or stabbing. Pay particular attention to the way the patient holds her body. Jennifer was grabbed by the left arm and thrown against the door before she was raped. It is important to be aware of the possibility of head trauma. (Jennifer's mood swings and unusual behavior may suggest head trauma.) If the mechanisms of injury seem apparent, these should be noted.

Interact

One of the first challenges you face in assessing a rape victim is getting permission to assess and treat. In large part, success may reflect the attitude that you bring to the situation. Three important principles are summarized in Box 6–4.

First, if you meet the victim at her level of distress, emphasizing compassion and a desire to protect, rather than to expose, you may overcome some resistance. An overprotective EMS provider may not allow the patient to initiate the normal process of working through her feelings. Meeting the patient at her level of distress is the first principle for involvement. It will also apply in other cases with victims of intentional violence. The treatment system should not repeat, even in a mild and well-intentioned way, any of the insults suffered in the attack itself. Violence has depersonalized the victim; being victimized reduces a person's ability to make decisions. Of course, the victim may have suffered some physical injury that will affect consciousness or decision-making

BOX 6–4

THREE PRINCIPLES FOR INTERACTION WITH A RAPE VICTIM

1. Meet the woman at her level of distress.

   Do not order her about.

   Do not overprotect her.

2. Emphasize your capabilities.

3. Allow the woman the time to reach her own decisions, if her injuries do not require immediate treatment.

ability, but the treatment process should bring in the victim as a partner to the fullest extent possible so that she is not robbed of further **autonomy.** You must reassure the patient that there is no danger of a subsequent attack. Your presence reinforces the fact that she can be helped and that you are part of that process. It is critical to stay with the patient throughout the intervention.

The second principle is to concentrate on your professional strengths. Your role is to treat and transport the patient. It is not to apprehend a rapist or to collect physical evidence from a crime scene. However, EMS providers should be able to perform their duties without confusing an investigation. Your ambulance service should have policies and procedures for such situations.

The third principle is that unless there are signs of serious physical injury, caring and compassion are more important to a successful outcome than speed.

Ask

There are a number of important facts that must be known in order to treat the patient successfully. You should be supportive rather than inquisitive or accusatory. Your inquiry should emphasize your concern with two immediate questions: "Where do you hurt?" "How can we help?" Vigorous questioning can take on the character of another assault.

It is important to know what medications the patient has been taking. A patient on a blood-thinning medication may be susceptible to bleeding problems. Do not overlook the possibility that the patient might have been pregnant at the time of the rape. However, it might be advisable not to raise this question specifically.

It is also important to ask the patient if she has bathed, washed, and changed clothing, or urinated after the assault. All of these actions have an impact on evidence collection and will be important to note on your reports as well as on the police reports.

Act

Vital signs should be obtained as soon as possible for a baseline measure and to assure that physical functions are stable. Treat any bleeding, sprains, or fractures. Administer oxygen as appropriate. A gynecological examination should only be done in the ED.

Every ED will follow rape treatment protocols. You should be familiar with these protocols in order to explain the forthcoming treatment process if required and to coordinate your care with that which will be given at the hospital.

Attend

Be supportive. It is important to be there, rather than focusing on getting the patient somewhere else. It is important that the survivor make her own decisions and regain control over her life.[4]

Document

The key to effective documentation is to report what is necessary for the patient's treatment, without revealing personal data unnecessarily. The victim– patient may say a great many things in the post-trauma period. She may be inconsistent, vengeful, suspicious. These are normal reactions to victimization. Extensive or vivid quotations are not necessarily helpful here.

However, your records may become part of a legal investigation, and some findings may be relevant in court. Your service should have policies and procedures for cooperating with police at scenes of crimes and safeguarding evidence. It is important that you know them.

 CONSIDERATIONS FOR EMS PROVIDERS

Senseless violence has a profound impact on helpers as well as direct victims. Working with a patient such as Jennifer Collins reinforces an EMS provider's own sense of vulnerability. Rape or assault can occur to anyone. After attending a victim of violence, you may share some feelings of vulnerability. There are healthy and unhealthy ways to deal with these feelings.

EMS providers, like police officers, may become cynical. If unchecked, this callousness may result in ineffective care. Remember that the victims may need to feel secure in order to accept a helping relationship. An attitude that sees the victim as just another statistic, rather than as a thinking, feeling individual in her own right, undermines this.

It is also important to be aware of your prejudices. Jennifer Collins was clearly an innocent victim. However, you may encounter situations in which the victim is a prostitute or a drug user. A professional response demands that these patients receive the same type of approach: nonjudgmental and respectful. Any victim should be given the opportunity to make decisions as appropriate.[2]

CONCLUSION

The consequences of rape can stay with the survivor for years. What you do in the minutes after the assault can help in the process of healing.

REVIEW QUESTIONS

1. How might a victim of intentionally inflicted trauma react differently from a victim of unintentional trauma?
2. List at least three reasons why a rape victim might not want to report a crime.
3. Identify at least three emotional reactions that a rape victim might experience.
4. List at least three reasons why a rape victim should have a medical examination.
5. Why is it important that a rape victim make her own decisions to the extent of which she is capable of doing so?

EXERCISES

1. Have a rape survivor address your group and report what he or she experienced.
2. Discuss why men rape women.
3. Discuss whether or not a rape victim should actually resist her assailant.

REFERENCES

1. Rape, Abuse, and Incest National Network and Bureau of Justice Statistics, U.S. Department of Justice. www.rainn.org/statistics.htm and www.ojp.usdoj.gov/bjs.
2. Clark, S. (1988). The violated victim. *Journal of Emergency Medical Services,* 13 (3), 48–51.
3. Hafen, B. Q., & Frandsen, K. J. (1985). *Psychological emergencies and crisis intervention.* Englewood, CO: Morton Publishing.
4. Los Angeles Commission on Assaults Against Women. (1982). *Surviving sexual assault.* New York: Cogdon and Weed.

FURTHER INFORMATION

Internet Resources

Sexual Assault and You: www.healthy-dating.com

National Clearinghouse on Marital and Date Rape: http://members.aol.com/ncmdr/

Rape Abuse & Incest National Network: www.rainn.org

Media Resources

Movies

The Accused

Act of Vengeance

Silent Witness

Bastard Out of Carolina

Sudden Impact

Books and Articles

Foa, E. B., & Rothbaum, B. D. (1997). *Treating the trauma of rape.* New York: Guilford Press.

Frank, E., & Stwart, B. D. (1984). Depressive symptoms in rape victims. *Journal of Affective Disorders, 1,* 269–277.

Groth, A. N. (2001). *Men who rape: the psychology of the offender.* New York: Perseus Book Group.

Nutt, D., Davidson, J. R. T., & Zohar, J. (Eds.). (2000). *Post-traumatic stress disorder: diagnosis, management and treatment.* Boston: Blackwell Science.

Wilson, J. P., Friedman, U. J., & Lindy, J. D., (Eds.). (2001). *Treating psychological trauma and PTSD.* New York: Guilford Press.

CHAPTER 7

The Brutalized Child
A Family in Despair

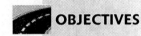

OBJECTIVES

Upon completion of this chapter, you should be able to:

- Describe the signs often associated with physical abuse in children.
- Explain the complications of working with the family of a possibly abused child.
- Demonstrate effective patient interaction.
- Understand the responsibilities of the EMS provider in effective treatment in child abuse.

THE CHALLENGE

A frustrated mother strikes her 2-year-old daughter who is tugging and pulling at her mother's skirt while she takes care of an infant brother; an angry stepfather beats his 9-year-old stepson who "mouths off"; a **distraught** father hits his 3-month-old daughter to stop her crying. The stories are common. Every year in the United States almost one million children suffer physical abuse, mental abuse, or neglect.[1] Confronted with abuse, or possible abuse, you face a triple challenge. First and foremost, you must protect and care for the child. This protection may involve bringing the case to the attention of social services if you are mandated reporters. Even if you are not **mandated reporters,** you should make sure that the emergency department knows of the possibility that abuse has occurred.[2] Second, you must recognize the needs of the parents or caretakers. Often they are far from sadistic monsters—they have frequently been victims of parental abuse themselves. Many are trapped, overwhelmed with guilt and fear. Third, you must treat yourself. Abuse can disturb even the most street-savvy EMS provider.

 ## THE PATIENT AND THE SITUATION

Three-year-old Wanda Jackson is rooting through the trash. This is the third time she has pulled the cover off the trash bucket to search for lost treasure. To Wanda, the bits of paper, old makeup tubes, and empty bottles are rare finds. To her mother, it seems as if Wanda is going out of her way to torment her. "Why are you doing this to me? You little terror. Go watch the cartoons for a while and let me get some sleep. You'll get it when I get out of bed." Wanda pouts briefly and then resumes her explorations.

Priscilla Jackson, Wanda's mother, faces another long, nothing day. She is hung over from the party last night. Her mouth feels like cotton. Her head aches and every movement is a reminder that she stressed her body with too much alcohol and too much dancing. She was first awakened by a call from her

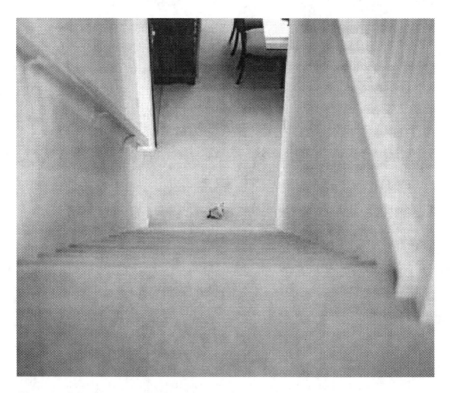

(Photo by Evan Richardson of Fortissimo Photography)

mother, who "just wanted to say hello" but ended up chastising Priscilla for her laziness, her drinking, and her stupidity for staying with Billy. She feels trapped, but, unable to confront this feeling, she drinks. She blames Billy, Wanda's father, for her pregnancy. She blames Wanda for keeping her at home. She blames society because she cannot get a job that will pay her substantially more than Wanda's day care would cost. Bleary-eyed, she looks toward Wanda. She says to herself, "If it weren't for you, I'd have finished high school and gotten a good job in an office."

Billy works occasional construction jobs. He says that they'll get married when he lands a full-time job with Mr. McNamara, the contractor. This is unlikely, however. Billy's Monday morning absences have pegged him as unreliable. McNamara has made up his mind that he will not hire him on subsequent jobs. Billy's relationship with Wanda is limited. When Priscilla nags him, he will grudgingly hold Wanda or give her a cookie.

After a few minutes of watching "Tom and Jerry," Wanda returns to her trash bucket treasure hunt. She smiles brightly as she goes after a red-and-white beer can in the bottom of the bin. Innocently, she brings the shiny bauble to her mother in bed, leaving a trail of stale beer along the linoleum. Priscilla screams. Rising quickly, she slaps Wanda's behind with her open palm. Wanda wails at the top of her lungs. Priscilla strikes her again—this time on the left shoulder—for crying. Priscilla screams, "Why are you doing this to me?" She knows Wanda can't answer. Priscilla vaguely realizes that this is what her mother used to say to her when Priscilla was beaten as a child.

For Wanda, the morning's slapping does not seem particularly menacing. She has been struck regularly by both Billy and Priscilla since she was born. Sometimes she was hit very hard; once hard enough to fracture her wrist. Other times, she was slapped sharply to "give her a message." There was an accidental scald when Wanda pulled a pot of boiling water off the stove, and there were several falls down stairs while Wanda was playing unattended. As an infant, Wanda did not attend a well-baby clinic, and she is not seen by a pediatrician.

When Billy comes home at noon, Wanda is happy to see him. Billy, however, doesn't want to see anyone. He is angry and frustrated. McNamara has told him he doesn't need him any more on this job. Wanda greets him at the top of the stairs. In his frustration, he pushes her aside too roughly. Wanda loses her balance and topples down the stairs.

In the seconds after his open hand pushed Wanda away, Billy's attitude changes dramatically. His anger gives way to disgust at himself. Priscilla sees Wanda at the bottom of this stairs. "My baby . . . my baby!" Billy calls 911. "My daughter fell down the stairs. She's not moving." He gives the address. The dispatcher repeats the address and asks Billy to stay on the phone while he dispatches the police and an ambulance. Then he gathers additional information. From Billy's description, he senses that Wanda's injuries may be serious. Priscilla wants to comfort Wanda, but a well-meaning neighbor warns her about moving someone with a possible broken neck. This advice terrifies Priscilla even more, but she publicly announces, "She just slipped. She'll be all right." Mentally she adds, "Won't she?"

The police, who arrived first on the scene, immediately immobilized Wanda's head and neck to prevent any further injury. Her angulated right ankle suggests a possible fracture.

Elizabeth Porter and her partner Jim Bateman had an uneventful morning. The dispatcher's order to proceed to Nevada Street for an unconscious child with possible head and neck injury has changed that. A crowd has gathered outside 20 Nevada Street. The EMS providers quickly brush through the onlookers and enter the hallway of the Jackson home. Wanda is lying motionless on her back at the foot of the stairs, the police officer's large hands holding her head and neck firmly. She stares at the ceiling. Jim and Elizabeth introduce themselves to Billy and Priscilla "on the run." Elizabeth finds out that the child's name is Wanda and that she is 3 years old. Elizabeth says gently, "Wanda, we are going to help you." Wanda does not answer. However, from the movement in her eyes, they know she is alert to voice. Jim notes that her right ankle is twisted at an abnormal angle. When Jim palpates it, Wanda sobs, "Go away! No! No!"

They place Wanda on a pediatric board. Elizabeth explains what they are doing in words she hopes Wanda can understand. Jim notes a large bruise on her left forearm that seems to predate the fall down the stairs. Wanda's pulse is thready at 124. Her blood pressure is hard to obtain but seems to be 140/80. Her respirations are irregular at 18. "I want Mummy and Daddy," she sobs. Elizabeth encourages Priscilla to calm her daughter.

As they work, they ask Priscilla for some basic information.

Priscilla asks, "Is she going to be all right?"
"We're doing everything we can for Wanda, Mrs. Jackson."

Elizabeth asks, almost reflexively, "What happened?" Priscilla becomes flustered. She starts to point toward Billy but catches herself. "She slipped. She was playing and she slipped. That's all."

Carefully collared and boarded, with her leg splinted, Wanda is readied for transport. Jim explains that they will take her to St. Francis Hospital, which has excellent services for children. They ask Priscilla to ride with them in the ambulance. Wanda screams, "I want to stay here."

Although Jim and Elizabeth have been schooled in nonjudgmental response, the scene is a disturbing one. They suspect that this incident was not a simple accident. First, Jim noticed a number of old bruises, including some that could have been cigarette burns. Second, the severity of Wanda's injuries did not seem consistent with a simple fall. Jim has a strong negative response toward suspected abusers. He thinks most deserve prison. He had no trouble in filling out the mandated reporting forms required by the Department of Social Services. Elizabeth had no sympathy for abusers, but since her daughter was born, she could understand how frustrations could build up. Before Amy was born, she could not understand how anyone could strike a child. She discovered that even a loving mother could find herself with a short fuse when cooped up alone with a colicky child for a long time. She wondered how a single mother could ever cope. She wondered how she would cope if it were not for her child care options.

THE PATIENT'S WORLD

Three types of people live in or around the abusing home. First, there is the child victim. An abusive home is often the only world they know. Second, there is the abuser or abusers. All too often abusers come from a background of abuse. Finally, there are the enablers. They often know what is going on but turn a deaf ear or respond ineffectively. They may be bound by their own fears.

Most often, the behavior that launches the abusive response is normal, age appropriate behavior. These behaviors may be misinterpreted by the parents as a challenge or insult. They, in turn, meet the supposed defiance with an act of physical retribution. Childhood is a series of new ventures. As the child succeeds in each of these ventures, he or she moves toward greater independence. This is normal development; it is not a conscious affront to parental authority. Psychologist Erik Erikson believes that the challenge for a child of Wanda's age revolves around autonomy: developing initial success in mastering physiologic processes such as toilet training and feeding. If the child does not master these functions, or if a child is constantly berated or belittled, he or she may develop a sense of shame and self-doubt.

In a few instances, the child may be extremely active and display a great deal of energy. Keeping up with such children can pose a real test of parental tolerance. However, their **hyperactivity** is not simply a means of provoking parents. It may have a physiologic habits.

Wanda is engaged in typical 3-year-old ventures. She searches her environment. She does not yet fully appreciate her mother's concern that garbage stay in the garbage can. She doesn't understand her mother's violent rage. If the pattern continues, Wanda may mature in a violent world. She may come to see nothing wrong with being hit. In a habit pattern, she may even expect periodic assaults.[3] She can adjust her life to realities. Her parents will dress her in long sleeves. She will choose not to invite friends over after school. She may adopt a pose of silence in front of teachers and friends to avoid disclosure of family secrets. To reveal these secrets would be disloyal and disrespectful.

Priscilla considered herself a good mother, despite occasionally losing her temper. She definitely did not view herself as an abuser. After all, she reasoned, children need discipline—especially strong-willed ones like Wanda. She knew she loved Wanda, but she did have her doubts about Billy's concern. Her fears grew as he postponed marriage, began drinking more heavily and more regularly, and worked less frequently. She didn't like his treatment of Wanda, but she feared saying anything. He might really walk out then. This was a double trap. She had to be responsible for Wanda, and she felt she couldn't ask Billy to take more responsibility. Yet, she never believed Billy would do what he did. She told herself repeatedly that Wanda slipped. But in her heart she knew Billy had pushed her first. She is uncertain which story to tell.

THE BEHAVIOR OF THE PATIENT

Wanda is afraid to tell what happened on the stairway. She thinks anything she says would mean being disloyal. She initially remains mute. In other cases, a child victim may tell what happened, but often it will take a long time to develop a trusting relationship. Even in a confident, trusting relationship, it is difficult for children to talk about what happened to them. Sometimes the child will openly describe what happened, only to deny it later.

The parents, or other abuser, can usually describe what happened but may be unwilling to do so, especially if a story must be corroborated with the other parent. A person who tells the truth doesn't have to remember what he or she says; a person who lies must. Quite often, the abuser will be concerned with what might happen to the child. This concern may be quite genuine.

A number of factors contribute to child abuse: economics, family stresses, drug use (especially alcohol), personality issues, and personal experiences.

Although child abuse occurs in all classes, economic stress is a fertile breeding ground for abusive behavior. People living on limited or tightly stretched incomes have few options and opportunities. Priscilla, for example, could not afford day care or baby-sitting services. Her poverty contributes to her sense of being trapped, feeling isolated, and seeing no options.

A family under stress, from whatever source, may turn on their child. Battles between parents may claim the children as casualties. Billy's interactions with Priscilla are often dictated by his work situations. His feelings about losing his job may be most easily transferred to Wanda. Severe sibling rivalry could result in aggression against the weaker child. Struggles between parents and grandparents can show up as conflicts in child rearing, resulting in the parent reacting strictly and forcefully with the child.

Drug abuse and alcoholism also provide fertile grounds for abuse. The drug-affected parent is already in diminished control of his or her emotions. Challenges, or perceived challenges, may elicit a disproportionate response. Prolonged abuse may result in significant organic problems that can affect the parent's ability to relate to a child.

Certain personality types may also tend toward abusive behavior (Box 7–1). Four are worth noting. First, the person with **ideas of reference** may personalize the meaning of behavior inappropriately. He or she may see the child as willfully disobedient or challenging. Second, persons who feel easily over-

---

BOX 7–1

FOUR PERSONALITY TYPES OF ABUSERS

1. Persons with ideas of reference
2. Persons who feel easily overwhelmed
3. Perfectionists
4. Persons who were themselves abused as children

---

whelmed and unappreciated have difficulty in caring for and nurturing a child. They may even look to the child to take care of them by doing small tasks and running personal errands. When this does not happen, they become frustrated, angry, and annoyed with the child. Consequently, they may get back at the child through violence or verbal abuse. Third, some parents, teachers, and clergy have an overly perfectionistic approach to the world. They demand correct, precise behavior and become punitive when standards are not met. Fourth, victims of parental aggression may inflict aggression on their own children. Child abuse passes from generation to generation within families.

 ## THE EMOTIONS AND THOUGHTS BEHIND
THE BEHAVIOR

Two emotions dominate the affective landscape of the abused child: chronic sadness and blunted feelings. Despite Wanda's involvement in exploring the garbage can and her apparent fascination with the beer can at the bottom, she often feels sad. Such a sadness is often the result of being battered and beaten. People, especially strangers, see despair and fear in her face. This sadness may persist into later childhood and adulthood. The emotions outlive the immediate pain.

Emotional bluntness is the second major affect. Teachers, friends, and daycare workers might note a certain reserve in a child such as Wanda. They perceive something lacking in her and in her interactions with others. A certain spirit is missing. She seems to maintain a distance from others.

These results can occur simply on the basis of psychological abuse. However, physical abuse—especially head trauma—can lead to a physical basis for problems such as these.

Following any injury, a child might appear shy and awkward around strangers. Even if physical scars heal quickly, scars in the thinking process can persist for decades. These result from the child's attempts to make sense of her parents and the world. Rollo May[4] notes that these effects may be far more severe in middle- and upper-class children who are indoctrinated with constant lessons about the basic goodness of parents and the stability of the family. A child lacks the ability to put parental mistreatment into its proper perspective. There is a very strong danger that the child will not develop a stable, positive image of herself.

In fact, many battered children incorporate into their self-concept the idea that they were responsible for the battering. They may think that on some level, they deserved it. Wanda's mother hit her. Wanda comes to see herself as a person deserving to be hit. She develops the following line of thought. "My mother hit me. I must deserve to be hit. Bad people are punished by being hit. I am bad."

Another basic thought pattern seen in victims of childhood violence is the inability to love or trust. One line of argument would go, "If I am bad, how could anyone love me?" This may be followed by "I cannot be trusted. I can't trust my instincts to tell me when I am going too far. I will go too far without realizing it. I need to depend on other people to set limits for me." From this, a beaten child comes to anticipate blame and punishment.

FAMILY/BYSTANDER RESPONSES

Abusers may be rich or poor, educated or uneducated, religious or without any faith. It is dangerous to stereotype the abuser. Such a stereotype limits an appropriate assessment of the child and his or her situation.

However, certain patterns may be seen frequently. Some abusers will hit the child for every perceived infraction. Violence dominates family interaction. Children learn and adjust to it. A contrasting pattern is the abuser who engages in episodic abuse. This pattern is often found among alcoholic and substance-abusing parents. For instance, an alcoholic father may come home and be very physical some days, hitting his children over small, insignificant bits of behavior. On other days, he might come home, shower the children with love and attention, and give presents. Still others, like Billy, in the case we described, become abusive around a major setback or adversity. They displace their anger onto their offspring.

An abuser may experience a range of emotions before, during, and after a hitting episode. Often a parent, teacher, or child-care worker feels anger, frustration, or even rage prior to striking a child. In other cases, the abuser may act not out of anger but out of a deep depression over perceived losses. Still other abusers may react to their own anxieties and fears. One parent of a 3 year old beat the child relentlessly after the child, who had been lost in the woods, was found safe and well. She screamed at the lad, "You made me worry."

During the violent episode, the abuser may experience a number of reactions. Some experience a sense of distance from the physical punishment. They are emotionally detached despite being involved physically. Others see themselves as righteous avengers armed with the conviction that the child deserved the punishment. Still others are overwhelmed with a sense of disgust. A few may be responding to internal stimuli such as hallucinations and delusions.

After the violence, a number of responses are possible. Guilt and remorse are common. Billy changed his attitude from, "the kid needs it," to one of guilt for inflicting more harm than he intended. Some will develop an amnesia for the entire interaction. Still others feel justified that they have set the child right.

Abusers often show thought patterns that justify their violence. Many come from the "spare the rod, spoil the child" school. They have a rigid view of discipline and frequently believe that children should be seen but not heard. They often lack age-appropriate expectations for the child. They will demand that a 2 year old have the attention span of an adult. Priscilla thinks that Wanda should be able to play all morning in one section of the room all by herself.

Many personalize the child's behavior and see it as aimed at "getting to" them. Perhaps Priscilla saw Wanda's resistance as a direct challenge and a bold act of defiance. She could not permit herself to see any other explanation, such as 3-year-old curiosity coupled with a short memory for parental injunctions.

Many parents resort to violence despite their own long-held beliefs that they would never hurt a child. Frequently, these people are themselves victims of abuse. Priscilla had glimpses of her mother's words and gestures as she struck Wanda.

Commonly, child abuse continues to exist because it is ignored by the community. Neighbors, friends, and teachers may have deep feelings that something is wrong, but they may fail to act on those feelings. Some will fear retribution; some will believe that "It's none of my business." Some will feel that they do not know what to say or do and hold back, hoping that things will get better.

In the days following Wanda's "accident," many people will admit to suspecting that something was wrong at 20 Nevada Street. A man who lives next door will remember hearing Billy yelling and Wanda crying at all hours of the night. Another will remember that Wanda frequently could be heard screaming shortly after Billy arrived home. Priscilla's mother always felt that Billy was no good. She frequently told Priscilla that she didn't trust him and now will tell all her friends, "But, my daughter wouldn't listen to me." She knew her daughter was in trouble but was powerless to help because of their strained relationship.

Clinic doctors and nurses, Priscilla's welfare caseworker, and the pastor of the church Priscilla attended before her pregnancy all had seen or heard of the abusive situation but were either too busy to do anything about it, lacked hard evidence, or were rejected by the Jackson family.

PROVIDER RESPONSES

As Elizabeth and Jim head toward Nevada Street, all they really know is that a child has been injured. They fear the worst but hope for the best. They are more concerned when they see that a police car is at the scene. They see Billy's agitation, Priscilla's confused attitude of concern and wariness, and Wanda's injuries, and they suspect abuse. Jim and Elizabeth know that they must report suspected abuse.

Each is saddened by the event and shocked by the abuse that likely preceded it. Even the most hardened EMS providers may experience a silent rage. They may seek explanations and look to legal or social procedures for retribution. They may carry a grudge into their next interaction with an abusing parent they encounter.

Some EMS providers, like some police officers, will see the abuser as worse than a criminal. They see the abuser as a person who has violated a special trust. They may treat the parents as guilty at the scene and spend time eliciting information that will punish the abuser. They may ask accusing, provocative questions of the parent or the child. They will move to protect the child from the villain. They will discount the parents' feelings.

Others may professionalize the whole situation. They will tell themselves that yes, it happened. The child and the parents both need professional help. However, it could never happen among the people I know, and I could never do such a thing.

Still others may ponder the enigma of abuse. Elizabeth Porter could not help but wonder how Priscilla felt as they took her daughter to the emergency room. She knows that if criminal charges are brought, the legal system will fail both Wanda and her parents. She knows that the press will deal with the situation in black-and-white terms.

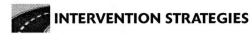 **INTERVENTION STRATEGIES**

Observe

In cases of suspected child abuse, EMS provider observations at the scene can be crucial. A quick look around an apartment or home will indicate if it has been child-proofed. The presence of electric socket covers, gates on stairs, and secure drawer closures indicate that the parents have a concern for their child's safety and health. Such safety measures suggest that the parents have a realistic view of a child's behavior. A clean apartment with an adequate supply of food suggests that children are not chronically neglected. However, these conditions in themselves are no guarantee that caretakers are not abusive.

The opposite conditions—especially if poisons, knives, or guns are within easy reach—may raise suspicions about parental concern. Of course, this does not indicate abuse, but, at the least, suggests negligence.

If a child has fallen, his or her location after the fall or the pattern of bruises and injuries may suggest abuse or support the contention that the fall was an accident.

Ecchymosis and/or scarring—especially in unusual locations—may indicate physical maltreatment. Similarly, unexplained burns should raise your index of suspicion. However, an injury that seems to be disproportionate to the amount of force described by the parents or others is not necessarily abuse. Children with diseases that result in brittle bones or who have blood disorders that result in excessive bleeding can be mistaken for victims of abuse. An appropriate history can uncover such factors.

Observe the interactions of the child and the caretakers. A child who exhibits fear of a caretaker may be the victim of abuse. However, this is not always the case. In some instances the child may gravitate toward the abuser due to the child's need to please the abuser. Such behavior can give the EMS provider a false impression of the relationship between the caretaker and the child.

Interact

Parents are deeply concerned. Keeping the parents involved and informed (as appropriate) can make a difficult situation better. In many states EMS providers, along with nurses and physicians and others, are mandated reporters of suspected cases of child abuse. Reporting suspected abuse to the appropriate authorities can prevent later tragedies. However, EMS providers should not make an issue of this during the initial interaction.

Ask

Your tone is as important as the choice of questions to ask. A temperate, nonjudgmental voice can ease a situation that may be hostile or at least suspicious. If the ambulance has been called by a person other than the caretaker, some defensiveness is not unexpected.

Taking a thorough history of the child is important but often difficult. Particularly if abuse is involved, the parents may not be cooperative, and an abused child may be guarded in talking with outsiders. Young children are poor reporters and may have a limited grasp of cause and effect. A parent under the influence of alcohol or other drugs may have an amnesia for the event and may be unable to clearly describe what happened. It may be worthwhile to ask about well-baby clinic or pediatrician visits. The answers to these questions can help you to gauge the health consciousness of the parents. Abused children often have little contact with medical services, except in emergencies.

Act

The role of the EMS provider is immediate emergency medical care and support. EMS providers are not trained social workers or police investigators. An inquisition of the parents or veiled accusations are clearly unprofessional. However, eliciting information directly related to the injury—especially information that may suggest hidden or past injuries—is appropriate. Likewise, paying attention to signs of abuse in your physical examination is appropriate. Look for such signs as loose or missing teeth, burns of mouth or tongue, bruises about the eyes, and deformity of the ear due to repeated trauma (sometimes called **cauliflower ear**).[5]

Wanda, like any victim of possible abuse, deserves medical attention first and foremost. However, there are a number of other important steps as well. First, as with any patient, never leave the child unattended. Your presence, once you have established rapport, can be comforting. As well, you may protect the child from further abuse. Second, do not make the situation worse by trying to enlist the child as a witness against a parent or other abuser. Leading questions concerning abuse or mistreatment can poison a situation. Third, listen to the child. Listen to her version of events. Despite cruel treatment, she may deeply love the abusing parent.

Attend

An EMS provider who takes time to listen will sometimes glean important information that questioning would never reveal. It is especially important to recognize that the parent may also be hurting.

Document

Good documentation can make the case for follow-up treatment of the child and his or her parents. Report claims and facts about injuries objectively. Your description of mechanism of injury as described by patient or caregiver should be included in documentation. Do not make prejudicial remarks that cannot be substantiated.

 CONSIDERATIONS FOR EMS PROVIDERS

EMS providers must discuss what happened. With appropriate regard for patient confidentiality, it is essential to clear the air. While treatment may be straightforward, working with the parents can be stressful, especially when it appears obvious that they are covering up the true cause of injuries. EMS providers should discuss the situation and their emotional responses with others who know something about child abuse.

Abuse also raises issues of legal or ethical reporting obligations. While state rules may vary, EMS providers have a clear obligation to the patient, which must include appropriately passing on information about unsafe or dangerous conditions. In-service education should fully familiarize EMS providers with their ethical and legal responsibilities in cases of suspected abuse.

CONCLUSION

Even if the injuries are not life-threatening, child abuse is one of the most difficult scenes an EMS provider can encounter. The family dynamics may make it difficult to treat and transport the child who is the patient. Yet, your attention to details can be critical in the care of the child.

REVIEW QUESTIONS

1. List two types of situations that might precede an incidence of abuse.
2. How does an abuser's own upbringing influence his or her child-rearing methods?
3. How might a history of abuse affect the self-concept of an abused child? How might it affect the child's relationship with the abuser?
4. What four personality characteristics may be seen in abusers?
5. What factors might make it difficult to obtain an accurate chief complaint or description of the present incident?
6. How should EMS providers approach the parent(s) of a battered child?
7. Why is good documentation important?

EXERCISES

1. Have an adult discuss with your group what it is like to be a victim of child abuse.
2. Have a rehabilitated abusing parent describe to your group both causes for the abuse and the treatment.
3. Hold a group discussion on ways to discipline children.
4. List factors that contribute to child abuse.

REFERENCES

1. National Center for Victims of Crime. www.ncvc.gov
2. Beebe, R., & Funk, D. (2001). *Fundamentals of emergency care.* Clifton Park, NY: Delmar Learning.
3. Miller, A. (1990). *For your own good: hidden cruelty in child-rearing and the roots of violence* (3rd ed.). New York: Noonday Press.
4. May, R. (1989). *Love and will.* New York: Bantam Books.
5. Perkin, R. & Van Stralen, D. (2000). 20 things you may not know about pediatrics. *Journal of Emergency Medical Services, 25* (3), 38–42, 44–46, 48–49.

FURTHER INFORMATION

Internet Resources

American Academy of Pediatrics: www.aap.org

Child Abuse Prevention Network: http://child-abuse.com/

National Clearinghouse on Child Abuse and Neglect Information: www.calib.com/nccanch/

Media Resources

Movies

Sybil

Schindler's List

Mommy Dearest

When a Man Loves a Woman

A Boy's Life

Books

Bass, E., & Davis, L. (1994). *The courage to heal: a guide for women survivors of child sexual abuse.* New York: Harper Perennial.

Lew, M. (1990). *Victims no longer: men recovering from incest and other sexual child abuse.* New York: Harper Collins.

Nutt, D., Davidson, J. R. T., & Zohar, J. (Eds.). (2000). *Post-traumatic stress disorder: diagnosis, management and treatment.* Boston: Blackwell Science.

Wilson, J. P., Friedmen, U. J., & Lindy, J. D. (Eds.). (2001). *Treating psychological trauma and PTSD.* New York: Guilford Press.

CHAPTER 8

The Potentially Violent Patient

Anxiety, Ambivalence, and Aggression

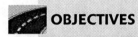 **OBJECTIVES**

Upon completion of this chapter, you should be able to:

- Understand basic safety measures that you can take when confronted by a potentially violent patient.
- Explain the importance of teamwork.
- Demonstrate safety skills throughout the intervention.
- Explain the ways in which the presence of families and bystanders can complicate an effective response.

THE CHALLENGE

The potentially violent patient is one of the most difficult of all psychiatric emergencies for EMS providers. Not only might the patient harm himself but also family members, neighbors, and people who try to help. Many EMS providers have not received formal training in managing violence and should defer to persons who are trained. If there is a potentially violent situation, the EMS provider must be accompanied by public safety officers.

It is necessary to understand the origins and dynamics of the aggressive stance in order to match the treatment to the patient, the situation, and the etiology. The challenge is not simply to maintain an effective treatment approach and transport if indicated but also to use your emergency medical care skills to minimize the danger of harm to yourself and others.

THE PATIENT AND THE SITUATION

Twenty-year-old Bud Brothers paces back and forth across the living room in his dingy, poorly lit third-floor apartment. His girl friend, Sheila Hardsworth, holding their 14-month-old daughter, Kimberly, stands out of the way near the kitchen. She is scared, terrified for her boyfriend's health and her and their daughter's safety. She called 911 5 minutes ago at 4:50 P.M. She told the operator that her boyfriend "was acting funny on his medications and she was afraid for her daughter and herself."

Sheila also wonders if Bud might have been drinking some beers. Their private but not too funny joke was that 'beer do not make Bud wiser.' In fact, alcohol of any type often made him angry and menacing.

When she arrived home with Kimberly she had found Bud staring vacantly at the wall. She assumed he was having an adverse reaction to his medication. Then, Bud started raving, pacing, and shouting "this goddamn world." It was then that she dialed 911.

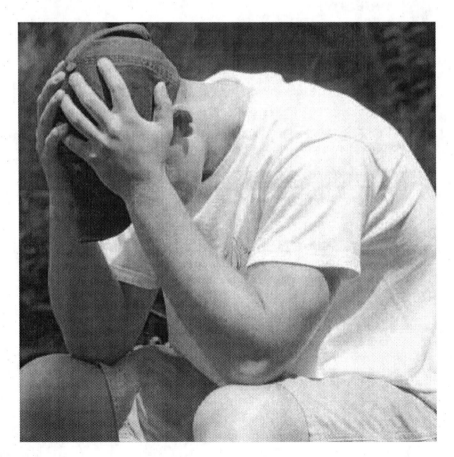

The dispatcher recognizes both the medical emergency and the potential violence of the situation. She notifies EMS and the police.

"I can't get a job. Do you give a damn?" he screams out the window. Sheila cares but does not dare speak for fear he might hit her again, as he did after she told him she had called for help. She wants to run to protect her baby, but she doesn't want to leave Bud alone. "That shrink don't know how the hell I really feel. Screw it, I know more than she does."

Sheila loved Bud's spontaneity and his freewheeling outlook on life but was deeply concerned when this dark side of his personality showed forth. He had come from a violent, broken home and he had vowed that *his* family would be different.

Unfortunately, it isn't. He dropped out of high school at age 17 and has been in trouble with the law twice: once for vandalism and once for driving under the influence of amphetamines. He had (and lost) six jobs in the 3 years since he left high school. Two years ago he suffered a concussion in a single-vehicle automobile accident. ("But it wasn't my fault. It was that bastard in the 'vette," he would explain as he described the episode.)

Bud paces the room with clenched fists shouting "nobody cares!" "Why can't they understand?" Sheila sobs, "I do care. I want you to work everything out." The door bell rings, startling Bud.

During the 5 minutes, which seemed like an eternity to Sheila, police car 31 of the Newtown police department with officers Frank Malone and Fred Jones sped toward the apartment. Also Unit 2 of Newtown's EMS service with EMS providers Bill Hallet and Marie James were en route. The two vehicles were in radio contact as they moved toward the scene. The EMS service had agreed to meet in front of the neighboring apartment house.

When the police officers and EMS providers arrived they greeted each other warmly; they had worked together in many situations before. Although Marie was particularly concerned about the patient's medical condition, Bill reminded her of the potential for violence and that an injured EMS provider would not help that patient. They decided that the police would enter first and then the EMS team. If the situation were to become violent, the police would intervene. If the patient appeared to be medical, then Marie and Bill would take the lead.

Officer Malone rings the bell.

"Who's there?" Bud shouts into the speaker. "I'm Frank Malone of the Newtown police with two EMS providers. We received a call to come to your apartment." Bud replies, "Go away pigs! I don't need help. Everything is fine up here."

Officer Malone explains that there had been a call and he cannot leave without seeing what is going on. "Hey, we only want to help." Bud again feels defeated and with a sigh of resignation reluctantly presses the buzzer. The two officers followed by Bill and Marie file up the stairs to the third-floor apartment.

Officer Malone knocks on the door. Sheila with a look of fear and amazement sees the group as she opens the door. Bud threatened her after the doorbell rang. But then he had become suddenly afraid and markedly tired. He moved away from her and slumped into a big, old comfortable easy chair. Sheila indeed felt that maybe Bud had been affected by his medication.

Sheila cautiously welcomes the group as she shows concern about her boyfriend's health. The two officers observe Bud and beckon Bill and Marie to advance, as they move over to the kitchen area to wait and watch.

Bill and Marie slowly, deliberately step toward Bud. He mutters, "What the hell are you doing here?" Bill identifies himself and Marie as EMS providers and states that they are concerned about his health. Bill points to his equipment kit. He says, "Mr. Brothers I would like to check your pulse and blood pressure."

Although Bud is angry with Sheila he recognizes that there may be something wrong with him. He also registers the fear in Sheila's face as Marie slowly moves her into the kitchen. He also is fully aware that there are two police officers standing near his kitchen and realizes he is in enough trouble. Yet, he is a proud person and feels he failed his family.

Bud starts to explain that he had taken some Valium prescribed by his family doctor, Dr. Ben Jones, for his low back pain and also his antidepressant from his shrink, Dr. Beth Wilder. He sobs, "I don't have a job and have not served my family well." Almost as though to undo that statement, he starts to clench his fist and wants to pace again. Bill responds in a concerned but firm tone, "Mr. Brothers please sit down and let me take your blood pressure and pulse."

Again, reluctantly, Bud sits back down and Bill tells him that he will be taking his pulse. Bill moves close slowly, reminding Bud that there may be something medically wrong with him. Bud pays a great deal of attention to the procedure. Perhaps he wonders if there is indeed something medically wrong. Bud's pulse is 144.

Meanwhile, Marie comforts both Sheila and Kimberly. Marie assures Sheila that she has done the right thing by calling 911. When Bud started to get up, she moved between him and Sheila and the daughter. Marie took a quick glance over to the officers and was glad they were there.

Suddenly, Bud feels angry and tenses up. He feels an internal fear and wants to run. He has run all his life. He really wants to strike out at the world and run. Bill senses and sees the tension and backs off. He recognizes the danger but also sees that Bud is not running. Simultaneously, the two officers take a step into the room. Bill signs with his hands that the situation is okay.

As quickly as the tension began, it now recedes. Bill states quietly, "This is a difficult time for you." Bud nods and suddenly feels connected and heard.

Bill explains again that he will now take Bud's blood pressure. Bud slowly offers his arm. Bill puts on the cuff and pumps it up. The blood pressure reading is 100/50. Bill tries not to show all his concerns. He states that he would like to check Bud out in the emergency department (ED). Bud is hesitant and worried. He asks if Sheila can come too.

Bill elects to use a chair to bring Bud down the stairs. Again Bud reluctantly, but with assurance from Sheila, accepts.

The police officers actually accompany the group and help carry the stair chair down the stairs.

 ## THE PATIENT'S WORLD

The agitated, potentially violent patient's behavior is characterized by activity, sudden movement, and loss of control. The predominant emotions are anger, fear, and apprehension. Underlying these emotions and behaviors is a view of the world very different from yours. The violent patient views the world of others with suspicion and mistrust, often attentive to, and attaching significance to, details of speech and behavior that others consider ordinary. Simple actions may be construed as threatening; a caring approach may be interpreted as a danger to be fought or as a signal to flee.

 ## THE BEHAVIOR OF THE PATIENT

For a potentially violent patient, the object of aggression may be walls, desks, cars, or people. The force used may range from fists to bottles to knives or guns—any handy object.

A variety of actions may precede an assault. The first **(prodromal)** period is marked by a gradual buildup of emotion. Between anger and rage may come an array of shouts, threats, mutterings, and epithets. Pacing and gesturing may increase. The enraged person may stare and glare at the helper. Often, his behavior is **paradoxical:** he may cry out, "Leave me alone!" while continuing to provoke and demand attention. A violent person will display a strong sense of territoriality, the need to control his space. If the patient does erupt into violence, that eruption is very abrupt and frequently devastating. From where does this aggression flow?

 ## THE EMOTIONS AND THOUGHTS BEHIND THE BEHAVIOR

Several strong emotions dominate the inner world of the violent patient. Two of these are especially important: anger and anxiety. Anger is born of frustration, loss, jealousy, or perceived injury. In some people the angry affect gives way to rage. For some, anger coexists with depression. Some people find this inner sadness hard to express. It is easier for them to express anger than grief. Despite the tough poise that violent patients may exhibit, they often wrestle with deep, inexpressible fears. For a great many individuals, aggression and assertion mask inner fear and uncertainty.

Anxiety—free-floating agitation—distorts the patient's perceptions and responses. Many patients who experience unfamiliar symptoms will show mild anxiety. If the patient cannot afford health care, this may significantly increase anxiety about seeking treatment. Moderate or severe anxiety is marked by agitation and may lead to violence. Anxiety may show itself in cold, clammy skin; rapid heart rate; distractability; or a general inability to engage in adult conversation. The severely anxious patient may completely lose control.[1]

Potentially violent patients may view the world as against them. They have a basic mistrust of others. They scan the environment with a heightened sense of vigilance because they fear attack. They often think in black-and-white terms, remaining quite stubborn, believing that, "If I give in on this point, then all is lost." They are frequently self-centered, demanding attention, "I want it now, now . . . now. Do you hear me?"

Two forms of psychotic thinking may dominate the potentially violent person's mental processes. These are delusions and hallucinations. Delusions are false ideas held against all logic. Delusions of persecution, such as the idea that the KGB, the CIA, the FBI, the Mafia, or a former employer are after them, may be paramount in their reasoning. These delusions may lead them to believe an attack is imminent and to launch the first strike. Delusions of jealousy lead to thoughts of betrayal and revenge. Delusions of **grandiosity** may lead the patient to believe that he is God and that if others do not obey his commands, he must punish them.

Hallucinations are false sensations that are perceived by the patient as real. The classic situation involves auditory hallucinations. The patient hears voices that are not there. Visual hallucinations also occur. A person suffering hallucinations can become violent when the sensations take on a commanding character. Hallucinations can differ. In some hallucinations the patient is ordered to commit a violent act. One **schizophrenic** patient reported that "voices in my head are telling me to kill my mother." In other cases, a patient may become violent to escape hallucinations. A 40-year-old man withdrawing from alcohol saw an army of angry women (a visual hallucination) bearing down on him. He knocked down several people attempting to flee.

Sometimes a violent patient is manic; that is, he or she suffers from a psychiatric syndrome involving irresponsible behavior, increased activity, grandiosity, and/or flights of thought. Manic individuals may have lost insight into the actual inappropriateness of their behavior.[2]

Why is Bud violent? Why has Bud attacked his girlfriend and now threatens even more harm? Two answers emerge: one is immediate and one is long-range. In this situation, Bud reacts to the loss of his job, his resultant depression, and the relaxation of inhibitions due to alcohol. However, a wide array of factors and environmental circumstances predispose toward violence. These include family background, past experience with stresses, medical history, **self-medication,** and substance abuse.[3]

There are a number of common threads in the histories of violent patients. As children, they have often witnessed violence in their homes and were victims of parental aggression (see Chapter 7). They have school histories that include tantrums and truancies. Their driving records often reflect impulsivity and difficulties with alcohol. Many have histories of losses in early childhood, such as the death of a parent.

Certain medical situations may promote violent behavior. Some patients may react to a diagnosis of diabetes or heart disease with anger and flight. In some pulmonary diseases, such as asthma or chronic obstructive pulmonary disease (COPD), aggression may emerge as a response to the feeling of breathlessness. Central nervous system injuries, tumors, encephalitis, temporal motor epilepsy, and head trauma have all been correlated with violence.

Similarly, a number of medications are known to promote violence. These include L-dopa, used to treat Parkinson's disease, and steroids, which are used in a wide range of illnesses. In some circumstances, antidepressants have propelled schizophrenics into more delusional behavior and manic-depressive patients from depression to violent mania.

Many substances either potentiate or precipitate violence. Alcohol is responsible for increasing aggression in many situations. It is a central nervous system depressant that reduces inhibitions and facilitates the expression of emotions that are typically held in check. Hallucinogens such as LSD, mescaline, and psilocybin can trigger a violent bad trip. Amphetamines, cocaine, and phencyclidine (PCP) are all associated with violent behavior.

Finally, some settings and some groups of people are associated with violent behavior. For example, in a motorcycle or youth gang some violent behavior is tolerated and even rewarded.[4] Of course, if weapons are valued in the group, this increases the probability that they will be available and used.

 ## FAMILY/BYSTANDER RESPONSES

Sheila kept her distance from Bud, protecting her daughter from what she recognized as a real threat. However, she also sought help for Bud and did not leave even when the opportunity presented itself. This is typical of the dilemma that the family of the violent patient faces. Families find themselves having to decide whether to flee or to help. On the one hand, they are terrified for their own safety. They feel fear, dread, and terror. On the other hand, because the cause of the pain is not an abstract stalker or a stranger in the night but a loved one—a spouse, a parent, or a child—they feel for, want help for, and identify with the predator.

The family may feel responsible for the violent behavior, that they have provoked the episode. Far too often, a suspicious individual provokes his or her family. In desperation, the family react negatively to accusations or taunts, which causes an outburst.

The common response of the family to violence remains fear. They have been threatened, battered, and broken. This fear gives rise to inconsistent, but equally attractive, alternative solutions: fleeing, fighting, or remaining stock still.

Emotionally, responses range from denial to sympathy and from revenge to identification with the aggressor.

 PROVIDER RESPONSES

The EMS provider is not only called on to apply his or her skill and training to a challenging patient care situation but also faces significant personal risk as well. As EMS providers weigh the potential benefits to the patient and the potential risks to others involved, they may question their own careers, their interest in helping others, and their own values. Like the family of the potentially violent patient, the EMS provider may wish to be elsewhere but be kept at the scene by a sense of duty.

The violent patient may trigger three different reactions in EMS providers. Some become angry in response to the patient's hostility and provocations and may wish to strike back, especially when the patient attempts to use physical force. Others may see the outward aggression as a manifestation of deep and painful troubles. Others may find themselves repelled and may treat the patient with an icy indifference. Rest assured that no one remains neutral when confronting a potentially violent patient.

 INTERVENTION STRATEGIES

Violence toward EMS providers is an important concern. Violence is particularly critical when it occurs in situations in which there is little reason to expect it. Do not rule out the possibility of violence based on the dispatch information.[4] Certainly if the caller is agitated, or threatening, violence is a strong possibility. In such cases, you should have police backup or other appropriate support. However, some callers will not give any indication of violence. Our example—a possible medication reaction call—gave no indication of potential for violence. However, Mr. Brothers' reaction when the EMS providers arrived could have been sufficient cause not to proceed without backup. There may be other cases in which there is even less of a clue from the dispatch information.

Observe

Before approaching the patient, you must survey both the environment and the patient. If there is a possibility of violence, check the patient and the immediate vicinity for any weapons or objects that might be used as weapons. These will include bottles, brooms, ashtrays, and other more obvious weapons such as guns and knives. Second, assess the patient for any signs of anxiety: agitation, inability or unwillingness to maintain eye contact, and general lack of composure. Obvious signs of disarray or visible wounds that may have been self-inflicted are danger signs. Third, examine the scene for any indications of drug or alcohol use that might exacerbate the situation. Bud's supply of beer might be a factor in his behavior. Fourth, scan the environment for possible escape routes for yourself and the patient.[1] Just as you do not want to be cornered, you do not want to corner the patient into a situation in which he or she will feel it necessary to fight for a way out. These important observational measures are summarized in Box 8–1.

Interact

A potentially violent patient may actually seek help and appreciate the need for assistance. However, if he feels he is losing control of the situation, he might strike out. It is perfectly natural to fear a violent or agitated patient. It may be appropriate to let the patient know that he appears agitated or anxious.[3] Sometimes it may help to let the patient know that you are apprehensive; in others it may be best not to show your concerns. Approach the patient slowly. Both your body language and your statements should be nonthreatening and nonjudgmental. "You look very nervous and upset. I can see you're wringing your hands. There's something going on here, and I'm here to help you."[1] Begin with relatively neutral questions.[5] It may or may not be advisable to offer a handshake. One of the traditions behind a handshake is that it is supposed to indicate that neither person has a weapon or intends any harm. However, it is essential to maintain a body buffer space. If you are too close, you might increase the patient's apprehension. Generally, keep yourself several feet away from the patient. Most people in our culture like to maintain a personal space of at least 4 to 6 feet around them. In public spaces, people may become sensitized when a person approaches within 12 feet.

The family's attitudes and level of supportiveness for the patient can give you important information in planning your response. In the story of Bud and

---

BOX 8–1

FOUR IMPORTANT OBSERVATIONS

1. Look for possible weapons in the environment and on the patient.

2. Observe the patient for any signs of anxiety such as agitation, unwillingness to maintain eye contact, and general lack of composure.

3. Look for any indications of drug or alcohol use that might affect the patient's emotional status.

4. Look for possible escape routes for yourself, the patient, and others, if necessary.

Sheila, Sheila was an important ally, supporting the EMS provider's position that Bud should get help. Bill and Marie also recognized that Sheila's absence might arouse Bud's anxiety. In other circumstances, it might be necessary to keep the family away from the patient. Generally, it is a good idea for the family to accompany the patient to the ED. In some cases, a family member might ride in the ambulance; in others, in their own vehicle.

Select one person who will be responsible for dealing with the violent patient. Others should be visible to the patient but far enough away that they do not pose a threat. Too many people on scene can cause the patient to feel overwhelmed and confused.[3]

Adopt a slow, deliberate, unhurried cadence. The patient may be highly sensitive and overly concerned with who is in control of the conversation. If the patient perceives you are moving too quickly, and thus are taking too much control, he or she may cut the interview short.

Offer the patient a choice of topics. In the introduction, the patient will probably identify a number of concerns. "Would you rather tell me about your headache or your stomach cramps first?" Strive toward equal-level discussion. If the patient sits, sit at a distance. If he stands, stand.

Attempt to understand the patient's frustrations, and if possible, identify some points on which you might agree. In Bud's case, the EMS provider might talk about his boss and his job and suggest by tone and affect that the employer might have been unfair. However, avoid any indications that you share any of the patient's delusions or hallucinations.

Assure him that you will take care of his belongings. It may seem a small point, but concern for a patient's dentures and eyeglasses will reinforce your stated concern for his dignity.[5]

Finally, if unexpected changes occur, be sure to explain them to the patient.[6] For example, if you are diverted from the hospital to which you told the patient you were going, explain this change in plans and the reason for it. Some intervention guidelines are summarized in Box 8–2.

Ask

There are a number of important questions that you must consider. In your mind, the most important question is probably, Why is this patient experiencing these symptoms right now?[6] However, as a general rule you should not ask Why? questions. These questions can raise anxiety levels and put a previolent patient on the spot. Ask the patient if he understands what is happening, and reassure the patient that you understand he is anxious. Ask if the patient has any known medical illnesses and takes prescribed medications. For example, a 48-year-old woman complained bitterly, "I am trapped in this arthritic old body." Her physician started her on cortisone—a steroid. The cortisone greatly eased her arthritis but precipitated an aggressive, **paranoid** reaction. Where a medical cause for a problem may exist, it is especially helpful to focus on the medical aspects of the patient's problem. In the case of such a patient, you can

BOX 8-2

ELEVEN INTERVENTION GUIDELINES

1. Don't handle a violent patient alone.
2. Use all five senses in approaching and understanding the situation.
3. Slow things down. Time is on your side.
4. Convey an image of quiet reassurance.
5. Don't take angry statements personally.
6. Label emotional statements appropriately: "You sound angry."
7. Maintain eye contact.
8. Watch for nonverbal cues such as clenched fists, posture, and foot positions.
9. Never ask Why? questions. What? questions are less threatening.
10. Clearly state your expectations for appropriate behavior and define consequences of assaultive behavior before it occurs.
11. Reinforce positive behavior. Don't focus on the negative.

(Reproduced, in part, from *De-escalation Techniques* recommended by David Siddle, Ph.D.)

appropriately emphasize her need to see the doctor because of her medical condition. Many people are relieved to find that there might be a medical reason for their emotional distress.

Because a wide variety of drugs, illnesses, and experiences have been related to violent behavior, history is extremely important. Find out if the patient has recently used alcohol or other substances. It is critical to know not only if the patient is currently using alcohol but also if he or she has recently stopped using alcohol or other drugs, because violence is associated with withdrawal reactions (**hallucinosis** and **delirium tremens**).

Questions and answers provide a bridge between you and the isolated patient. Yet, for many paranoid patients, questions are an unwarranted intrusion. Hence, you must proceed with caution. It is important to ask nonjudgmental questions. Make inquiries from a respectful distance and allow the patient to maintain his or her own space.

Families can provide valuable data about a patient. Often because of the patient's belligerence or resistance to treatment, the family may be the only source of important information. Information should be gained from the patient if possible, but asking family members such questions as, "Has he been like this before?" "Has he any medical problems or is he taking any medication?" "Is there a substance abuse problem?" may provide critical treatment data.

Act

In the area of action, it is easier to identify inappropriate than appropriate actions. There are three things that you should never do.

First, never deal with an armed patient. If the patient is armed, the situation is a police matter. If the patient has either a gun or a knife, retreat and let the public safety professionals take control and command of the situation.

Second, never accept a weapon directly from a patient. If he has a gun, the situation requires immediate police-level intervention.

Never turn your back or leave the patient unattended unless this action is necessary to protect your own safety. If, for your own safety, it is necessary to leave the scene, do not return without police support.

The right things to do will depend on the situation, but there are three guidelines. First, explain what you are going to do and why. (The law or policy may require that he not walk to the ambulance. Explain that the safety belt is for his safety and comfort. If it is true, tell him that he will be out of the ambulance shortly.)[5] Second, do not assume that if you have been assaulted you need to answer with physical force. Keeping calm may be the best demonstration that you are in control.[5] Third, if it appears that force may be required, display your troops before threatening to use them.[7] Many violent patients, after surveying the environment, decide that a fight is unlikely to be successful and accept help.

The question of restraint is a thorny one. If you find that the patient requires restraint, have the police intervene. Beebe and Funk note that "A medically necessary restraint is ordered by a physician and done only for the safety of the patient or others" (p. 508).[8] Of course, a patient should be secured properly on the stair chair or stretcher. However, as an EMS provider you have no authorization to use formal restraining devices. If a patient is transported with police restraint, such as handcuffs, the officer must go with the patient in the ambulance.

Do not remove any physician- or police-ordered restraints, no matter what the patient says he will or will not do. Make sure that the inside of the vehicle remains free of potential weapons. An IV bottle or an oxygen tank can be a dangerous missile.

Attend

Paying attention to the violent patient is the key to a successful intervention. The paranoid patient continually scans his environment for signs of imminent attack and for indications that others are concerned about him. Not listening suggests a lack of interest. Listening shows respect and may tip the balance toward an acceptance of your offer of help. By paying attention to the patient, you may be able to detect early, subtle changes in behavior. Finally, do not leave the patient alone.

Document

Documented physical findings are very important. Vital signs will provide important information. For example, a patient going into delirium tremens often has an elevated temperature. Time of arrival, time at the scene, and time of arrival at the hospital provide important medical–legal documentation of patient care. If the patient is restrained, it is important to document the potential for or the actual escalation for violence that justified the restraint and to document that an appropriate humane technique was used.[7]

Quotes are especially important with the violent patient. A patient may alter his story or offer a completely different explanation at the ED (once he has had a chance to create "an alibi.") In one case, a belligerent, intoxicated 35-year-old man was found standing in the middle of the sidewalk, threatening to kill his wife. Later, in the ED, he denied having done this. The EMS provider documented his statements, helping the emergency physician to determine the best course of treatment for the patient.

The violent patient taken to the ED today may be a plaintiff in court action in coming months, charging the ambulance with excessive force, unauthorized restraint, or physical injury. Laws vary from state to state regarding who may be restrained and the restraint that is justified. Know the laws in your state and follow them. Excellent, detailed notes describing your intervention, explaining your actions, and recording observations about the crisis furnish the basis for good patient care and good legal defense.[9]

 CONSIDERATIONS FOR EMS PROVIDERS

EMS providers have twin responsibilities when dealing with a potentially violent patient. First, they must protect themselves and each other. Second, they must deal with the experience after the fact.

As we have emphasized throughout, you must protect yourself. You must be prepared to recognize the causes of violence and to recognize techniques that are likely to be effective in managing the violent patient. This instruction should include verbal skills and nonviolent physical techniques to parry an assault. EMS providers must keep constant vigilance. Too often, an attack occurs when it is least expected. When danger is anticipated, call for police backup. A potentially violent patient provides a test of healing skills, not of machismo.

An EMS provider who is threatened or physically attacked by a violent patient may suffer an indelible mental mark. The emotional trauma may be more devastating than the physical. It is difficult to integrate this experience into professional career experiences. It is critical to discuss these incidents, with the aim of understanding patient dynamics, EMS interventions, and emotional impact on the team. Many EMS providers will find the act of restraining or grappling with another individual very discomforting. The experience cries out for exposition, ventilation, and review.

CONCLUSION

It is important to treat all patients with respect. However, when there is a potential for violence, it is essential not only to keep yourself safe but also to work with local public safety officers and let them take the lead when indicated while rendering care.

REVIEW QUESTIONS

1. What are some of the factors that might lead a patient to become violent?
2. What can you do to protect yourself when assessing or treating a previolent patient?
3. What should you do if a previolent patient becomes violent?
4. How would the presence of lethal weapons alter your response to a potentially violent patient?

EXERCISES

1. Watch the movie *Natural Born Killers* and discuss whether this film or other media violence leads to aggression.
2. Discuss which films you would let your children watch.
3. Review factors that contribute to violence. There are a great deal of them.
4. What steps can you take to restrain a violent patient?

REFERENCES

1. Leisner, K. (1989). Managing the pre-violent patient. *Journal of Emergency Medical Services, 18* (7), 18–20, 23, 26, 28–29.
2. Soreff, S. & McInnes, A. (2002). *Bipolar affective disorder.* www.emedicine.com.
3. Hafen, B. Q. (1995). *Psychological emergencies and crises intervention.* Philadelphia: Prentice Hall.
4. Gilligan, J. (1996). *Violence.* New York: Vintage Books.

5. Soreff, S. (1981). *Management of the psychiatric emergency.* New York: John Wiley & Sons, Inc.

6. Parker, R. (2002). *EMS evaluation of psychiatric emergencies.* www.templejc.edu/dept/ems/pdf/ce%20Articles/PYCH.PDF.

7. www.the_mdu.com.

8. Beebe, R., & Funk, D. (2001). *Fundamentals of emergency care.* Clifton Park, NY: Delmar Learning.

9. Dernocoeur, K. K. B. (1996). *Streetsense: communication, safety, and control* (3rd ed.). Redmond, WA: Creative Options.

FURTHER INFORMATION

Internet Resources

Center for the Study and Prevention of Violence: www.colorado.edu/cspv

Minnesota Center Against Violence and Abuse: www.mincava.umn.edu

National Coalition Against Domestic Violence: www.ncadv.org

Media Resources

Movies

Once Were Warriors

Lord of the Flies

Natural Born Killers

The Unforgiven

Full Metal Jacket

Books

Benedek, E. P., & Cornell, D. G. (Eds.). (1989). *Juvenile homicide.* Washington, DC: American Psychiatric Press.

Soreff, S. M., & McNeil, G. N. (1987). *Handbook of psychiatric differential diagnosis,* Littleton, MA: Yearbook Medical.

Tardiff, K. (1996). *Concise guide to assessment and management of violent patients* (2nd ed.). Washington, DC: American Psychiatric Press.

CHAPTER 9

Depression and Suicide

A Semester in Hell

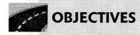 **OBJECTIVES**

Upon completion of this chapter, you should be able to:

- Understand the significance of depression and suicide in society and in your work.
- Explain how family members' attitudes toward the patient may change during the course of the illness.
- Demonstrate effective patient history-taking skills.
- Explain the importance of remaining with the patient at all times.
- Explain the importance of documentation as a part of a continuing process of care.

THE CHALLENGE

Approximately 9.5 percent of the U.S. population has a depressive disorder.[1] Depressed patients exist in a world of worthlessness, hopelessness, and helplessness. Their disease drains them and those around them. You may feel overwhelmed by a depressed patient yourself. However, you can provide necessary support to the patient and gather important information that will contribute to the healing process. Unfortunately, some EMS providers respond ineffectively—either by failing to grasp the seriousness of a depressed patient's situation or by inadvertently contributing to the landscape of despair.

Complicating EMS provider responsibilities is the fact that a depressed patient is at high risk for suicide. According to the National Institute of Mental Health, "More than 90 percent of people who kill themselves have a diagnosable mental disorder."[2] Many more attempt suicide but fail. A severely depressed patient may not be able to muster the energy to carry out a suicide attempt. The highest rates of suicide occur during initial "recovery" when the patient seems to be improving.[3]

The danger of self-destruction is greatest when the patient has a plan and the means to accomplish that plan. Even in the absence of a plan, a patient with the means of destruction at hand can be dangerous to himself.

The challenge to the EMS provider is to confront the depression, to face squarely the issue of suicide, and to intervene effectively to begin to reverse despair and prevent self-destructive behavior. Depression is treatable and suicide is preventable.

 ## THE PATIENT AND THE SITUATION

Twenty-year-old Billie Ann Small starts to pen a suicide note. She is sitting in her second-floor apartment in a wooden frame rooming house at the edge of campus.

> Dear Mom and Dad, Betsy, Tom, Irene, Jill, Joan, Joyce, Elizabeth and Susan,
>   April is the cruelest month. I feel overwhelmed, lonely, useless, empty, unsuccessful. I am a failure and a fool. I both regret and am glad that the end is near and peace is at hand. Please forgive me, but I have no one and you all have each other. I love everyone, but no one knows what I am going through. Some of you may wonder why I feel this way. . . .

As she writes, she wants to live. She wants to live as she sees other people living. But fearing that this is not possible for her, she wants to die. College is too demanding, her love life nonexistent, her attention span has decreased, and her grades have suffered. Billie believes she will fail most, if not all, of her courses. She is defeated by circumstances and feels publicly humiliated by her inadequacies. Billie has been drinking hard liquor regularly over the past 6 months to help her cope. Today she has taken many aspirin tablets. Her brother has a history of drug abuse and had attempted suicide once. Her mother has had bouts of depression, which are now controlled with an antidepressant. Billie Ann does not want a life like theirs; she sees no alternative but death. She has hinted to her friends that she might not be around too much longer. Lately, her closer friends have seen a change for the better. She seems more sure of herself.

Her friend Joyce Davis is still concerned for her. When Billie did not show up for her English Lit examination at 10 o'clock, Joyce was worried. Now, at noon, Billie failed to show for lunch. Joyce goes to Billie's room. At first, she gets no answer. Then she hears a rustling of paper. She knocks again, calling Billie's name.

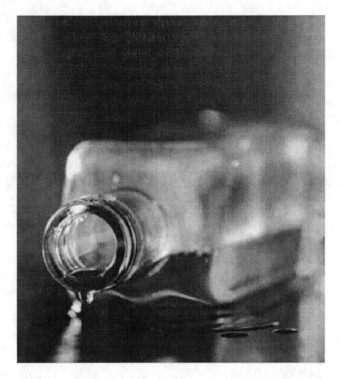

(Courtesy of PhotoDisc)

Billie sobs quietly and says, "Joyce, please go away now. I really, really don't want to see anyone." Billie speaks slowly. Her voice is muffled and somewhat slurred.

Joyce calls Mrs. Kane, the landlady, who knocks on the apartment door. No answer. Using her key, Mrs. Kane lets herself in. Billie is sitting, her head in her arms, breathing slowly and sobbing. Joyce smells the liquor and sees the note. "Mrs. Kane, call the ambulance! Something's wrong with Billie." Joyce walks Billie around. She's tried to sober up drunken boyfriends before. She holds the folk belief that walking around, hot coffee, and cold showers will help.

Mrs. Kane is not sure what is wrong with Billie but guesses, from her long experience with college students, that it is an overdose. Billie was such a good tenant, though. She never had any trouble.

The dispatcher at the fire station determines that Billie responds to verbal stimuli and is breathing, but she may have ingested some combination of alcohol and other drugs. He dispatches the ambulance for a possible overdose.

Rosemary Spencer and Jackson Walton receive the call and are en route within a minute. Rosemary is uncomfortable with overdose calls, especially if the overdose might have been intentional. In contrast, Jackson is intrigued. He has had a positive experience treating a suicidal patient and is anxious to help.

When they arrive, Mrs. Kane ushers them into Billie's apartment. Billie attempts to retreat toward the bedroom. Joyce blocks Billie's way. They introduce themselves, and Jackson asks, "What's happening?" Billie does not reply. Joyce states, in an overly loud voice, "She's been drinking and taking those pills," pointing toward a bottle of aspirin. Actually, Joyce does not know what pills, if any, Billie has taken.

Billie, shaking and sobbing, shouts at the EMS providers. "Get out. Go away. You don't understand. You don't care. And, there's nothing you can do anyhow." Jackson says, "You seem to be really overwhelmed. I'd like to help you." He leads her back over to the sofa. Billie says, "I can't keep up with everything. I'm a failure. I'm not going to be able to come back to school next semester, and I can't face my family after letting them down so badly."

Jackson says, "I can see why you might think everything is hopeless. It hurts to feel that you've let down your family." He adds, "Perhaps you're feeling very tired now? Your friend said you've been drinking and taking some aspirin. Is that right?" Billie says she does not know how many aspirins she has taken. "What were you going to do if your friend hadn't come by?"

"I have some sleeping pills."
"Have you taken any yet?"
"No, I needed to finish my letter."
"Have you ever attempted to harm yourself before?"

Billie hesitates for a second. She has not tried to kill herself, but she thinks of her brother who did make an attempt. She tells Jackson she has not, but her hesitation suggests to Jackson that there is more to the story. He does not pursue this line of inquiry but asks, "Can I check your pulse and your blood pressure?" Billie agrees.

While he takes vital signs, Jackson asks her about her family and friends. He restates his interest in doing what he can and tells her that he knows Dr. Gordon at the hospital has helped other people who felt that everything was hopeless.

Despite the note, the liquor, and the pills, Billie is ambivalent. She wants to die and she wants to live. Joyce's discovery of her suicide attempt and now the EMS provider's command of the situation actually come as a relief to her.

Jackson tells Billie they will be taking her to the hospital. She passively accepts. Her consciousness is fluctuating. They place her on a stair chair to take her to the ambulance. Both Jackson and Rosemary noted her warm skin and are concerned about how many aspirins she may have ingested.

As they leave, Mrs. Kane wishes her well, assuring her that her apartment will be there for her. Joyce accompanies them to the hospital.

THE PATIENT'S WORLD

A depressed patient dwells in a bleak, featureless landscape. Whatever the cause—cocaine withdrawal, alcohol abuse, loss of a spouse, loss of a job, a brain tumor, manic–depressive illness, internal voices becoming unbearable, or some physiological imbalance—the patient sees the world through gray-colored glasses,[4] experiences the overwhelming feeling that nothing will change for the better.

Suicide seems to offer the only way out. The decision to commit suicide may be followed by a relaxation of tensions, a new ease in relationships. The depressed person may appear calmer—as if she is getting better. The decision to commit suicide often leads to a sense of relief. However, some become more anguished in their relationships with family and friends. All depressed patients should be treated as potentially suicidal.

THE BEHAVIOR OF THE PATIENT

Three types of behavior dominate the picture of the depressed and suicidal patient. First, there are activity disruptions that accompany depression. Second, there are actions associated with a suicide attempt. Third, there are actual self-destructive acts.

Activity Disruptions That Accompany Depression

In depression, normal activities of daily living are disrupted. Some of these are summarized in Box 9–1. Sleeping, eating, and sexual disturbances are common. Some patients cannot get to sleep, and some cannot stay asleep. Others may sleep too long. These disturbances can be incapacitating in their own right and may accentuate the depression. Some depressed patients are starving themselves; others eat ravenously. Sexual activity can also tend to extremes: some patients

---

BOX 9–1

DEPRESSION-ASSOCIATED BEHAVIOR PROBLEMS

Sleep disorders	Oversleeping or inability to fall asleep or stay asleep
Eating disorders	Self-starvation or excessive eating
Sexual disorders	Loss of interest or hyperactivity
Interpersonal problems	Dependency or isolation

become hypersexual; others lose all interest. Isolation and alcohol use frequently accompany depression.

Depression can lead to two different patterns of interaction. Some people become dependent and clinging, totally overwhelming others. They refuse to be left alone. Others withdraw. They distance and disengage themselves from family and friends.

Some suicidal patients, especially patients who have been drinking, may become violent, suddenly directing outward the hostility they had been directing toward themselves.

Actions Associated with a Suicide Attempt

For a person becoming suicidal, seemingly disconnected events fit into a lethal pattern. The depressed person may stockpile medications. He or she may draft a will, may visit old friends, or write enigmatic messages. He or she may compose suicide notes, or purchase firearms. The case of one 45-year-old woman who believed she had inoperable cancer illustrates these activities. On the day of her overdose, she visited her church, said goodbye to her daughter and son, and went to see her sister.

Self-Destructive Acts

The means that patients may choose to kill themselves differ in their lethality, with guns being the most lethal. Some patients may combine two methods such as overdosing on sleeping pills and slashing their wrists.

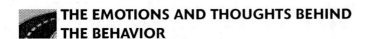

THE EMOTIONS AND THOUGHTS BEHIND THE BEHAVIOR

Dysphoria—overwhelming sadness—is the cornerstone of depression. Closely related to this may be anger—an anger that leads to thoughts of suicide as revenge. Billie's note, with her list of names, may indicate this scenario. The psychodynamic literature suggests that anger turned inward leads to depression and suicide. Anger turned outward may become aggression and violence.

Some depressed patients may feel tremendous inner turmoil. This turmoil may involve command hallucinations: voices that instruct the patient to kill herself. Other depressed patients may feel *nothing*. In one case, a 23-year-old woman with an extensive history of psychiatric hospitalizations slit her wrist as a way of gaining some feeling. She felt dead inside and wanted to experience any feeling even if it was pain.

Helplessness, hopelessness, and worthlessness pervade the thinking process. Depressed patients see themselves as incapable of being helped and beyond any intervention. These thoughts may be compounded by feelings of guilt for numerous past sins, which cannot be absolved. Life loses any sense of meaning. In fact, they see themselves to be of no value.

The thoughts that justify—even require—suicidal behavior are varied. Some depressed patients see themselves as so bad or so insignificant that the world would be better off without them. For others, self-killing is an act of revenge. Still others may see death as the means to reaching heavenly reunion with a loved one. Some suicidal thoughts appear as commands that must be obeyed. A person experiencing such a command hallucination may feel that she has no choice but to obey the directions given by voices within her head. These directions may include hurting herself or others.

Many roads lead to depression. It may be triggered by a loss for example—a death, a job or school failure, or a broken relationship. It may result from a chemical imbalance, as in manic–depressive illness. It may follow as a consequence of amphetamines or cocaine. Many medical diseases produce the symptoms of depression, for example, hypothyroidism, anemia, or pancreatic cancer.

Regardless of the etiology, once the patient has become clinically depressed he or she will feel overwhelming despair, as discussed earlier.

A number of factors correlate with suicidal behaviors besides depression. Alcohol abuse and intoxication have strong links to self-destruction. Billie's despair is intensified and potentiated by her drinking. A family history of suicide is a big risk factor. Other factors include chronic, debilitating, or terminal illness, or a history of incest or isolation. The feeling of being trapped with no alternative is an important cause. Suicide risks are also high in such conditions as schizophrenia and panic disorders as well as in depressive or manic–depressive illness.

How does depression develop? Initially, depression is an attempt to protect the individual—a defense mechanism. The depression represents one method of handling overwhelming loss in the outside world through retreat from the world, but the defense can fail. Suicide becomes a way of escaping the pain of depression.

 FAMILY/BYSTANDER RESPONSES

The family at first may react with sympathy to the plight of the depressed patient. They are sympathetic and caring and feel the patient's sadness. When the sadness continues despite their efforts at change, the family may adapt to it. They no longer empathize; they work around the depressed person as the family of an alcoholic may work around the alcoholic. Ultimately, the depressed patient may "burn out" the family. The family becomes angry, hostile, and distant.

When a depressed patient becomes suicidal, some families respond with support; others with indifference or rejection. Most families will respond to a first suicide gesture with alarm and concern. The same family may become indifferent to later attempts. One case, which continued over several years, illustrates this point. A mother, discovering that her 16-year-old daughter had taken several aspirins in a suicide attempt, immediately called the local rescue unit and her husband. Three years later when the same young lady, with a history of failure in school and work and several hospitalizations, took her fifth overdose, her mother reported simply that she was disgusted by her daughter and her problem. Some families even actively enable a suicide by buying pills or leaving them about, leaving the patient alone with weapons, or otherwise encouraging lethal action.[5] A depressed patient can wear down a family and a support system.

 PROVIDER RESPONSES

A depressed patient can exhaust EMS providers as well. Depressed patients can evoke a depressive response in those who try to help them. A patient who has suffered unfairly can draw the sympathy of most EMS providers, at first. However, if the patient continues to experience setbacks and to find no effective solutions, he or she can wear down helpers. For some EMS providers it may be difficult to separate professional responsibility from personal empathy. Other EMS providers may experience just the opposite reaction. They feel that the depressed patient should "pull up her socks, snap out of it, do something about her life." For such EMS providers it may be difficult for them to "walk a mile in the other's shoes." There is a middle ground, and that middle ground involves maintaining a professional, caring relationship.

Responses to a suicidal patient will also vary, depending on the EMS provider, the patient, and the circumstances. A suicidal patient may call out deep feelings of concern and empathy, especially if the losses leading to the attempt are ones with which an EMS provider can identify. For example, we know of one patient who lost his job when his company moved out of state. He drove his car into a tree. He sustained only minor injuries, but in listening to his story after the crash, the EMS providers felt anger toward the company and sympathy for the patient. This kind of sympathy is inappropriate if it supports the patient's self-destructive stance.

In other cases, the EMS providers will be clearly baffled by the patient's behavior. "He has a great job, good income, a beautiful wife, and two nice kids. Why would he want to commit suicide?" In other cases, EMS providers may express inappropriate, negative feelings toward the person who has made repeated gestures. For example, two EMS providers responded to a suicide gesture at the home of a depressed teenager who had made ineffective attempts at cutting her wrists four times previously in the past year. When asked why she had done it, she replied, "I felt like it. Now help me." The team felt a muted rage. They had just come from a call where several children had been seriously injured in a motor vehicle accident. One said angrily that he had "no time to listen to her stuff." Still other suicide attempts may elicit only apathy, "Oh, you did it again, eh, Joey." This response is probably most common with patients who employ suicidal gestures as a coping mechanism.[3,6] In these ways, EMS providers' responses can parallel those of the patient's family.

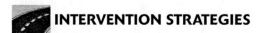 **INTERVENTION STRATEGIES**

Observe

The patient's environment may reinforce depression. Overcrowding, disorganization, filth, and lack of proper safety precautions should be noted. Remember that this is the environment to which the patient will be returning. If these conditions exist, they should be considered in discharge planning. You may be able to pass on important information to other members of the treatment team in this regard. More relevant to immediate emergency care, look for medications, weapons, rope, alcohol, or other devices that could be used in a suicide or in aggression against others. Your observations of conditions can make a difference. We know of one 62-year-old man who was mildly depressed. The EMS providers reported he was living in a dimly lit apartment with little food, a large collection of medicines, and a number of handguns. These observations led the emergency department (ED) physician to consider hospitalization for this mildly depressed patient whom he might otherwise have sent home.

A depressed patient may give physical cues to depression. Often he or she will be disheveled, unshaven or unwashed, with unkempt hair and dirty fingernails.

Determining whether an accident was really an accident or a suicide attempt may hinge on the presence of subtle clues. Often these clues are ones that you are in the best position to observe.[7] For example, one 22-year-old man took an overdoes of sleeping pills before driving his car into a bridge abutment. An alert EMS provider saw the pill bottle and brought it with her to the ED. Often, there is a suicide note. This note may give clues to method, as well as to motive, which might be important later in patient care.

Interact

It may be difficult to engage a depressed patient in conversation. The patient may not look at your face and may avoid eye contact. It may be useful to let the patient know that you recognize his or her sadness. "Ms. Small, you look very sad," tells the patient that her discomfort is apparent. Do not force attention on a depressed patient. It is probably best if one EMS provider takes the lead in interviewing and treating the patient. Be caring, but quiet. The depressed patient does not want to be told, "Pull yourself together!" or some equally domineering or belittling command. As one author notes, "When you are having a difficult time, do you look for someone who tells you how to solve every aspect of your problem? Or do you look for someone who will quietly allow you to talk it out?"[8] A patient may decide to confess shameful or criminal behavior to you. Perhaps this behavior is the stated reason for a suicide attempt. This is an awkward situation. Focus on the patient's feelings rather than judging him or her.

Ask

The more specific the threats of suicide and the more detailed the plans, the greater the probability of lethal, self-destructive activities. The potentially or openly suicidal patient can be confronted directly on this issue. "Do you ever think about ending it all?" "Do you wish it were all over?" The questions may sound as if they are putting ideas into a patient's head. In fact, the patient probably has entertained such ideas. The key is to ask the question without judging or punishing.[3] An important history question would be, "Have you ever attempted to commit suicide before?"[9] Rund suggests that a particularly dangerous pattern is one in which apparent lethality of attempts escalate with each subsequent attempt.[9] Follow up by asking, "How did you feel about surviving?" If the patient says he or she felt relief, the current risk may be lower. If, however, he or she felt angry or frustrated at being rescued, the risk may be higher.[9]

If a patient is contemplating suicide, these questions bring her concerns out in the open where they can be assessed and addressed. If a patient can describe a specific plan for killing herself in response to your question, "How would you kill yourself?" that person is at higher risk than one who does not have a plan. If the patient has the means at hand, the possibility of suicide is stronger still. A related question, "Is anything keeping you from killing yourself?" may identify sources of concern or strength that can later be tapped in treatment.[10]

Act

First and foremost, conduct a thorough physical assessment. A depressed, potentially suicidal patient may show signs of previous injuries, especially about the wrists. If there has been, or might have been, a suicide attempt, note the possible method and consider specific assessments that might be necessary. If a suicide attempt has involved hanging, pay particular attention to airway care. If an attempt involved slashed wrists, do not overlook the possibility that the person may have taken drugs as well. Vital signs will provide important clues, as will a standard mental status examination. Under no circumstances should the patient be left alone.[10] Someone must go to the bathroom with the patient if necessary.

In the ambulance, make sure that the patient is safe. Do not leave the patient alone. Equally important, make sure that the patient does not have access to syringes, or potential weapons, such as unsecured oxygen bottles. The patient must be secured for his safety and yours. For example, we know of one depressed 24-year-old who awakened after an overdose of alcohol and antidepressant medication. When he realized he was still alive, he tried to lunge for the rear door. Only the safety straps on the cot prevented a successful escape.

Attend

Do not assure the suicidal patient that everything will be all right. This assurance will ring false. It will seem to confirm to the patient how little you understand about his or her feelings. Instead, listen to what the patient has to say. Remember that suicidal crises are episodic. They last only several hours or at most several days. Survivors are glad they survived. The crucial intervention must simply be to keep the patient alive.

Document

We have already mentioned some important features of documentation. Describe the setting, the physical findings that may suggest prior attempts at suicide, any current physical findings related to suicide, level of consciousness, vital signs, and any changes during treatment and transport. Note any comments regarding the value of life or desirability of suicide that the patient offers.

 CONSIDERATIONS FOR EMS PROVIDERS

Depression leading to suicide or attempted suicide involves profound pathology. The behavior cannot be understood in everyday, rational terms. The reasons for the depression and the suicide attempt may be physiological, psychopathological, and interpersonal. The key point is that it is not for the EMS provider to look for or judge reasons for the behavior but to deal with the emergency consequences of it.

A depressed patient can be depressing. A suicidal patient who is well known can be frustrating. Recognize that the depressed patient is a deeply disturbed individual. One of the best ways to understand depressed patients is to read first-hand accounts written by survivors of depression. Every account emphasizes the utter hopelessness and helplessness that overwhelms the sufferer at the time of the depression.

EMS providers who have low self-esteem or a poor self-image may have difficulty understanding a depressed patient. An EMS provider who puts himself or herself down may find it difficult to hear the pain of a patient in depression.

If depression is a problem for you or your colleagues, it is important to recognize that prompt care can help. Depression and suicidal impulses are temporary and treatable.

CONCLUSION

Depression is sometimes called "the common cold of psychiatry." A patient with major depression may have "burned out" family, friends, and EMS providers. However, depression is treatable and persons who have contemplated or attempted suicide are generally glad that they did not succeed. Remember suicide is a permanent solution to a temporary problem.

REVIEW QUESTIONS

1. How might some of the behaviors associated with depression affect the patient's physical condition?
2. Does a depressed patient pose a possible danger to an EMS provider?
3. Why might the family of a suicide patient not be supportive of an EMS provider's efforts to help?
4. Is it appropriate to ask if the patient has considered suicide?
5. What can EMS providers do to reduce the likelihood that a patient will attempt suicide while in their care?

EXERCISES

1. Have a suicide address your group and have that person review the experience and express gratitude for the intervention.
2. What life experiences would make you depressed?
3. Visit an inpatient psychiatric unit. Observe and listen to folks; they have much to tell and teach.

REFERENCES

1. http://www.nih.gov.news/NIHRecord/05_2001/story08.htm
2. www.NIMH.nih.gov/research/suifact.htm
3. Hafen, B. Q. (1995). *Psychological emergencies and crisis intervention.* Philadelphia: Prentice Hall.
4. Soreff, S., & McNeil, G. H. (1987). *Handbook of psychiatric differential diagnosis.* Chicago: Year Book Medical Publishing.
5. Weissberg, M. (1983). *Dangerous secrets: maladaptive responses to stress.* New York: W. W. Norton.
6. Hafen, B. Q., & Karren, K. J. (1989). *Prehospital care and crisis intervention* (3rd ed.). Englewood, CO: Morton Publishing.
7. Barry, P. (1989): *Psychosocial nursing assessment and intervention* (2nd ed.). Philadelphia: Lippincott, Williams and Wilkins.
8. Soreff, S. (2002). Suicide. *www.emedicine.com*
9. Mitchell, J. T. (1995). Medic suicide. *Journal of Emergency Medical Services, 20* (11), 41–45.

10. Soreff, S. (1981). *Management of the psychiatric emergency.* New York: John Wiley & Sons.

FURTHER INFORMATION

Internet Resources

American Psychiatric Association: www.psych.org

American Psychological Association: www.apa.org

National Association of Mental Health: www.nmha.org

The 1999 Surgeon General's Report on Mental Illness: http://www.surgeongeneral.gov/library/mentalhealth/home.html

Media Resources

Movies

Dead Poet's Society

Girl Interrupted

I Never Promised You a Rose Garden

Ordinary People

A Beautiful Mind

Books

Copeland, M. E. (2002). *The depression workbook: a guide for living with depression and manic depression* (2nd ed.). Oakland, CA: New Harbinger Publishers.

Durkheim, E. (1997). *Suicide: a study in sociology.* Free Press, New York, NY.

Greive, B. T. (2000). *The blue day book.* Kansas City, MO: Andrews McMeel Publishing.

CHAPTER 10

Alcohol Abuse

Broken Bottles, Broken Dreams

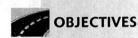 **OBJECTIVES**

Upon completion of this chapter, you should be able to:

- Understand the significance of alcohol and other substance abuse in society and in your work.
- Explain the dynamics of addiction and the behavioral consequences of acute intoxication.
- Explain what is meant by codependence and how it may affect family behavior.
- Identify appropriate ways to approach the person who has been using alcohol or other drugs.
- Ask relevant questions to construct a history and guide treatment.

THE CHALLENGE

The alcohol abuser may be seen by EMS providers as a nuisance and a danger rather than a challenge. The following bit of dialogue rings true in some services:

"How was your shift last night?"
"Kinda slow—only four calls, all just drunks. It seems as though I can't buy a real ambulance call."[1]

The challenge in caring for the alcohol-abusing or alcoholic patient is twofold: first, to look beyond the intoxication to conduct a thorough assessment, and, second, to maintain professionalism in a situation that can stress professional behavior to the limits. Intoxicated patients are often verbally abusive or at least unresponsive to EMS providers' questions. The intoxicated patient may present a physical threat to an EMS provider either because of the patient's loss of control over emotions of because of the patient's general inability to cooperate in treatment.

Alcoholism and problem drinking are pervasive, affecting between 10 and 20 million Americans.[2] As every EMS provider knows, alcohol is a factor in many injuries and medical conditions. It is a contributing factor in almost half of all murders, suicides, and accidental deaths, accounting for the loss of more than 100,000 lives per year.[2] Excessive alcohol consumption is the most common cause of cirrhosis of the liver, the third leading cause of death among adults between the ages of 25 and 59.[3] Most experts agree that alcoholism, defined by loss of control over consumption and withdrawal symptoms, is a disease that is treatable and arrestable but not curable. The disease is chronic and progressive, attacking the alcoholic physically, mentally, and spiritually.

Although this chapter focuses on alcoholism, the basic principles can be applied to treating patients intoxicated by other substances as well.

 ## THE PATIENT AND THE SITUATION

Wendell Phillips, 38, has been drinking steadily since he arose at noon on Sunday. The first two beers from his private refrigerator in his tool room relieved a hangover from the night before. The next six-pack accompanied a Chicago Bears game. Because he drinks beer, Wendell does not consider himself a "boozer." His wife complains about his drinking, but he says she has nothing to gripe about. He likes a few beers. It doesn't interfere with his work. Wendell has always been a good provider. He is a master electrician, and he never drinks on the job. He knows that alcohol and electricity do not mix. However, he has been refusing work in the past year. Some days he will not work beyond midafternoon. After the Bears game, he went out for cigarettes and stopped at his local bar, Foley's Tavern. After six more beers, Foley decided that Wendell had enough. Wendell washed down his last beer with a couple of painkillers the doctor had prescribed for a bad back.

After 14 beers in 5 hours, Mr. Phillips' blood alcohol level is over .02 ("point two" or two tenths of 1 percent). "Point one" is defined as legally intoxicated in most states. The Valium chaser has contributed to his intoxication in ways that he cannot begin to understand but that he does appreciate physically. To Foley, and the other patrons, Wendell is obviously unstable on his feet. Wendell thinks he is doing just fine. He feels great; he thinks he can conquer the world. As he leaves the bar, he misjudges the width of the doorway and bumps his left temple on the door frame. A few minutes later, he collides with a parking meter. At 5:00 P.M. on a bright fall Sunday, Wendell Phillips is sitting out on

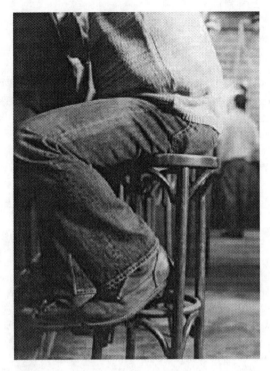

(Courtesy of PhotoDisc)

a bus stop bench, holding his right side, muttering indistinctly, and moaning occasionally.

A well-meaning passerby calls the police dispatcher, reporting a man in pain, speaking incoherently, sitting at the bus stop. The dispatcher asks, "Is he drunk?" The citizen reports, "He's had something to drink, but he doesn't look like a drunk. I mean a *real* drunk. I think he's sick." The police dispatcher refers the call to the municipal ambulance.

Roy Jones, age 44, a firefighter EMS provider for 20 years, and Tom MacLeish, a 20-year-old newcomer to the department, receive the call from the police with a decided lack of enthusiasm. En route Roy gripes about "another drunk call." He tells his famous story about the time that he picked up an old drunk with scabies and was out for 2 weeks.

Tom listens and feels that Roy speaks with the voice of experience, yet he is also bothered by Roy's view. Two events in his life have given him much to think about. His favorite uncle, Bill, a 44-year-old city police sergeant, was pulled off the streets and told that if he wanted to keep his job he would have to get help for his alcoholism. At first the family refused to believe that Bill could have done anything wrong and assumed that "someone was out to get him." However, Bill entered a 28-day residential program and came out of treatment with new optimism. Second, Tom had just seen an announcement of a new addiction treatment program at the general hospital. Tom thinks about these things, but as they approach Wendell, he is still not going to question Roy's wisdom.

The ambulance rolls up. A few passersby stop just within earshot. They are more curious than concerned and more observant than involved. Roy is relieved that Mr. Phillips does not look like a derelict.

Mr. Phillips greets Roy and Tom and then drops into an alcoholic fog. Roy responds, "How are you today?"

Roy is not sure why the ambulance was called. He suspects that there is nothing more than simple intoxication here—a police matter, if anything—but he attempts to do a thorough assessment. He notes a small bruise on Mr. Phillips' left temple: "Does it hurt you?" Wendell asks, "Are you police? What are all these people doing here?" Tom moves the small crowd back, hoping to disperse most of the rubberneckers. "We have the situation under control. We have a man with minor injuries. He'll be more comfortable if you stand back."

Wendell appreciated Roy's concern over his bruised head and Tom's dispersal of the crowd. He is feeling quite drowsy now. Roy bends his knees, bringing himself down to Wendell's level. He asks Wendell how he's feeling. Wendell says his stomach hurts and he doesn't want to go anywhere. "Where does it hurt?" Wendell points awkwardly to his right side. "When did it start?" Wendell has no sense of time and can only say that it came on before he sat down, while he was walking. "Let me see what I can feel." Wendell startles visibly when Roy palpates his rib cage about the 10th rib. There is no obvious deformity and no obvious mechanism of injury, but Roy suspects that Wendell has bruised or fractured a rib.

Roy completes a thorough assessment and finds nothing remarkable. He and Tom splint Wendell's right arm to his rib cage with a sling and swath and prepare him for transport. Just as they are moving Wendell onto the stretcher, Wendell looks up at them with a sheepish grin. Both EMS providers feel a warm sensation through their jacket sleeves and see a wet spot spreading around Wendell's pelvis. Roy and Tom think, almost in unison, "God, I love this job," but to their credit they hold on to Wendell and transfer him successfully to the stretcher.

In the ambulance, as Roy drives, Tom takes the opportunity to ask Mr. Phillips some questions. "What is your name, please? Where do you live? Do you know what day it is? Do you know where you are now?" Tom is not only showing concern and respect, but he is also evaluating Wendell's orientation to person, place, and time.

Wendell answers haltingly but apparently accurately. He tells Tom, "You remind me of my son. This is really great what you're doing for me. You aren't like those other no-good bastards." In fact, Wendell becomes highly sentimental when he drinks. He tells everyone who helps him that they're better than "those other no-good bastards."

THE PATIENT'S WORLD

The alcohol/substance-abusing patient is like a rudderless ship: out of control. This is true whether the abuser is a college student who has had too much to drink on spring break, a 45-year-old homemaker who drinks Bloody Marys for breakfast, or a 50-year-old binge drinking truck driver who goes on a bender once every few months. Occasional overindulgers put themselves and others at greater risk of injury, but they suffer few long-term consequences from intoxication itself. An occasional abuser may not know his limit, but he or she is not obsessed with the drug or alcohol.

Actively drinking alcoholics, in contrast, orient their lives around alcohol. Even if they are not continually grossly drunk, the alcoholic is concerned with securing, stockpiling, and consuming alcohol.

There is no typical alcoholic. The homeless derelict—"the poor unfortunate"—is simply the most obvious case. However, most alcoholics are not homeless—only 3 to 5 percent of alcoholics are.[4,5] In fact, most of the homeless are not alcoholics, but deinstitutionalized mental patients, persons with personality disorders, addicts of other drugs, and people whose basic problems are economic. Most alcoholics are employed, and professionals are overrepresented in the ranks of alcoholics. Doctors, nurses, dentists, and lawyers contribute disproportionately to the alcoholic population. What all share is a dependency on an addictive drug. Their addiction creates problems for those around them (codependents) who experience severe disruptions in their lives.[6]

THE BEHAVIOR OF THE PATIENT

Intoxicated behavior is inconsistent and erratic. Alcohol alters sensation and perception. Vision and hearing are impaired with high doses of alcohol. The eye requires a longer time to adjust when exposed to a very bright light. The ability to discriminate between sounds is reduced. The most significant effects in terms of behavior are on motor performance. An intoxicated person will sway when trying to stand steady with eyes closed. Reaction times are slower.[7]

An inebriate may be calm and curious at one moment and belligerent— even homicidal—the next. For a patient who is generally depressed, alcohol can bring him or her to the brink of suicide. In others, alcohol may trigger a grandiosity that leads to feats of great strength.

It is also important to realize that many inebriates will experiment with using other drugs along with alcohol. Some will routinely mix their drugs to attempt to achieve a desired high. Some drugs will have a synergistic effect, increasing the central nervous system effect of the alcohol.[8] Drug interactions pose a real challenge in assessment and treatment. Amphetamines and cocaine propel some to increased motor activity. Opiates and marijuana promote sedation and withdrawal from the world.

A person who is addicted is driven to obtain the drug to which he or she is addicted. Addicts experience physical withdrawal symptoms when they are without the drug. The alcoholic gets "the shakes" or auditory hallucinations, or, in especially severe withdrawal, delirium tremens. In addition, the addict suffers psychological symptoms in the absence of the drug: an obsessive desire for the drug and an overwhelming sense of insecurity or inadequacy. This extreme want becomes translated into drug-seeking behavior: hiding a secret supply; stealing to obtain the drug; neglect of personal, family, and work responsibilities; and, most inexplicable to a nonaddict, denying the addiction.

The illegality of a drug (alcohol for those below the legal age, and all controlled substances that are abused) leads the addict to secretive, even paranoid behavior. Wendell gulps down his pills, keeps a separate refrigerator in the tool room stocked with beer, and declines to talk about his experiences.

THE EMOTIONS AND THOUGHTS BEHIND THE BEHAVIOR

Wendell swings from despair to exultation and back. Alcohol is widely viewed as a stimulant because of its disinhibiting effects. In fact, its principal effects are as a central nervous system depressant. Alcohol relaxes feelings of self-criticism and inhibition. Alcohol also tends to increase risk-taking behavior.[7] In the sober person, intellect controls emotions; in the drug-affected person, emotions control intellect. The person may at one moment be caught in the depths of despair and at the next be "on top of the world." As the effects wear off, the user may "crash." The high becomes a low, marked by physical pain and guilt. During withdrawal, the patient may experience a tremulousness and **hyperreflexia,** which suggest that as the nervous system effects of alcohol (or other depressant drug) wear off, the system compensates by rebounding. The patient does not gradually come back to normal but experiences a wide swing to the agitated side of normal before settling down.[7]

Alcohol and other drugs alter a person's perceptions about himself, his destiny, and his world. Under the influence of a drug, a person may experience delusions, hallucinations, and **illusions.** These changes in thought process can have significant implications for any caregiver. For the EMS provider on the street, understanding these drug-affected states can mean the difference between rendering effective care and becoming a victim. Indeed, desired changes in thought and sensation are the reasons why many people begin using the drug. Alcohol and other central nervous system depressants reduce tensions; hallucinogens, such as LSD, alter the world of sensation. The effects of a drug vary depending on the substance, the mental set of the user, and the setting in which it is used.[9]

Finally, in a drug-altered state, a person may misinterpret the environment or may develop hallucinations. Mental images may appear to have an external reality (hallucinations). In other cases, ordinary objects may be seen as frightening apparitions. These are called illusions. For example, an intoxicated man believed a long, black object on the floor was a snake; it was his walking stick. During withdrawal from alcohol, auditory and visual hallucinations may occur during the first 48 hours after the person stops drinking.

When most people look at a drinker like Wendell Phillips, they think, "Doesn't he know what he's doing? Why does he do it? Why doesn't he stop?" The answer to the first question is that he may not know what he's doing. Alcoholics deny, minimize, and rationalize their behavior. This denial sounds extraordinary because the effects of intoxication are evident to the sober people around the alcoholic. However, in a drug-affected state, the alcoholic's ability to receive feedback on behavior is limited. Further, an alcoholic rationalizes the reasons for drinking, often blaming others for the sorry state he's in. "Anyone with a job like mine would drink." Even more inexplicable to a social drinker, an alcoholic may "black out." This does not mean "pass out," but rather it means that an alcoholic can continue to function and have no memory of what he or she has done. There are documented cases of alcoholics flying or driving to strange cities and having no idea of how they got there or why they went in the first place. Blackout drinking is one of the earliest signs of alcoholism.[10]

Why do alcoholics continue to drink? There are many reasons; most of them have nothing to do with the reasons why social drinkers drink. First, alcoholic— out of control—drinking may have a genetic basis in some alcoholics. It has been show in studies that, even when raised apart from natural parents, "children of alcoholics are more likely to have alcohol problems than are children of nonalcoholics."[11] Second, many alcoholics are physically dependent on the use of alcohol to make it through the day. They drink because they experience physical pain if they do not.[7] Third, the alcoholic is unable to function socially without alcohol.[10]

As to why Wendell, or any alcoholic, doesn't stop, the reasons may be very complicated. Initially, he may have begun drinking simply because it was expected in his social world. He may have progressed to drinking alone, or for the effect—to ease a sense of loneliness or inadequacy, or to provide a shot of liquid courage that helped him to deal with women or authority. He may have begun self-medicating, that is, treating a depression with his own bottled tranquilizer. After several years of addictive drinking, he may be drinking to satisfy a physical or psychological craving—to eliminate a pain that comes with any attempt to abstain. He may literally know of no alternative. He may be involved in a social world that expects him to drink. Of course, many drinking buddies are simply looking for social support and not for any true companionship or intimacy, but if this is the social world a person knows, it can be difficult to detach from it.

Many of the most successful programs, such as Alcoholics Anonymous, employ a 12-step approach to recovery. Successful rehabilitation requires radical changes that are difficult to achieve without strong social and emotional support. What many nonalcoholics fail to realize is that a "recovering" alcoholic who has worked through the recovery process becomes a far more mature and fulfilled person. Recovery is not simply stopping drinking but adopting of a whole new way of life.

 FAMILY/BYSTANDER RESPONSES

In some cases the family may support the need for detoxification or other medical treatment. In other cases, they may oppose it. Alcohol abuse leaves the family disabled. Quite often the family needs help as well.

Codependents, persons who are married to or deeply involved with alcoholics, and children of alcoholics have come forward to deal squarely with the problems caused by alcoholism.[6,12]

Families of alcoholics, like families of depressed patients, will vary tremendously in their response to alcoholic-related crises. Some families will unwittingly enable the alcoholic to continue his or her drinking by providing excuses and supports. Others will completely reorganize the family roles to meet family functions. In the case of a family with an alcoholic father, the mother may take on additional financial responsibilities and the oldest children may become "little mothers" to the younger ones. This family reorganization can leave deep psychological scars that last into adult life and affect the adult child of an alcoholic's own family life.[12]

When the intoxicated person is being assessed in public, bystanders may crowd around. This curiosity is inevitable. Some bystanders will be very sympathetic to the plight of the intoxicated patient and will be concerned that he or she is treated with consideration. This concern is also true of homeless patients, who may or may not be intoxicated. More serious problems in control arise when some of the bystanders are intoxicated themselves and have their own ideas about how the patient should be treated.

 PROVIDER RESPONSES

Many EMS providers, like police officers, treat the alcoholic or addict with a "cuff and stuff" approach. For many, a patient on a "bad trip" means that patient gets a quick trip. This behavior may stem from the sometimes mistaken belief that nothing is really wrong and that "the sooner this run is over, the sooner we can get a real ambulance call." It may arise from the concern that the alcoholic is an unpredictable and troublesome patient. The troubles range from odor and appearance to behavioral problems to limited control over body functions.

However, it may also arise from a deep-seated resentment of alcoholics and alcohol abusers. Such resentments are rooted in personal and professional history and are difficult to put aside. For some EMS providers, the alcoholic is a threat—a grim reminder that the pleasures of drinking have a dark side. There may be an unconscious desire to distance oneself from the failed drinker.

There are six different ways in which alcohol-abusing patients get involved with the emergency medical system. First, there are alcohol-related accidents, some of which are suicide attempts.[13] Second, there are intentional traumas resulting from drinking and inebriation: the barroom fight, for example. Third, there are alcohol-related illnesses, such as alcoholic hepatitis, cirrhosis, or **Korsakoff's psychosis** (short-term memory impairments and behavioral changes that occur without clouding of consciousness or general loss of intellectual abilities). Fourth, there are withdrawal-related conditions such as seizures or delirium tremens. Fifth, there is **pathological intoxication** in which a person exhibits bizarre behavioral symptoms after only a small amount of alcohol. Finally, there is inebriation itself, which can bring an abuser to the attention of both police and medical systems. Each of these conditions can be frustrating to the caregiver because the alcohol abuser is generally not a good patient.

These six ways point out the fact that each patient needs a thorough assessment and cannot be stereotyped. The medical system sees the alcoholic at his or her worst and poses a real threat—separation from the bottle. The alcoholic may also pose a more subtle threat to the EMS provider—especially the EMS provider who enjoys a drink. The alcoholic represents failure in a society that values alcohol.

 INTERVENTION STRATEGIES

Observe

Alert EMS providers can discover important information about the emergency and the patient that would otherwise be lost. First, do not assume that alcohol is necessarily the substance taken or the only substance taken by the patient. The scene will yield information about other substances taken, routes, and possibly amounts used. Reporting other known medications may alert the hospital for possible additive or synergistic effects. An empty cupboard or refrigerator may suggest that effects of abuse are coupled with malnutrition. A supply of knives, razors, or other potentially lethal tools may suggest a potential for suicide or aggression.

Interact

Remember that the alcoholic can only be psychologically evaluated when sober.[14] What Publius Syrus said nearly 2000 years ago is still true today: "To dispute with a drunkard is to debate with an empty house."[14] Cutting down on outside stimulation and distractions is an effective trick of the trade when dealing with an intoxicated patient.

Nevertheless, interacting with the alcohol-abusing patient requires a well-planned approach. The first few minutes can be crucial in determining the success of your intervention. The less commotion, the more likely your success. Remember that alcohol impairs the ability to adjust to change in the environment. The inebriate, once distracted, may be difficult to refocus on assessment and treatment. Further, he or she needs boundaries defined.

Begin with a firm orientation that clearly describes who you are, what you are there for, and the types of help that you offer. This can cut down on the patient's misidentifications and any paranoid thinking. Make it clear that you are not the police, and your uniform does not represent arrest. Do not use demeaning terms of reference such as "pops" or "Joey" or "dearie." Addressing the alcoholic by name may help with this orientation, as well as demonstrating a basic concern for his or her identity as a person.

Boundaries need to be set concerning physical safety, participation in the assessment and treatment, and moving to the ambulance. The EMS provider must be specific in describing what must be or will be done but flexible in recognizing that the inebriate's ability to respond is drug-affected. Standard precautions such as using latex or vinyl gloves should be taken.

Ask

Emphasize the physical concerns you are addressing. First and foremost you are assessing injuries and illnesses that need emergency care. Stress that you are assessing and treating the patient because of your concerns about his or her physical health. Reinforce your concerns by using stethoscope, blood pressure cuff, and penlight. Talk to the patient. Ask questions. The answers will help you to ascertain the inebriate's mental status. Ask questions about drug and alcohol use without being judgmental. A patient is often reluctant to describe use of illegal drugs or may be unable to explain exactly what he or she has taken. However, this is important clinical information in itself. Ask "What have you taken? When did you take it? How much have you taken? Have you used it before? For how long?"

Other preexisting medical situations may be exacerbated by the substance abuse. Relevant histories must include seizure disorders, mental illnesses, hypertension, and pregnancy.

The family may be able to provide information about the patient, the substances ingested, the history of abuse, and other relevant history. Remember, however, that the family's involvement may be very complex.

Act

The danger of being urinated, defecated, or vomited on is real enough that precautions should be taken. Beyond this, there are a number of simple, direct, and effective approaches in treating the alcohol-abusing patient. Obtain vital signs early in your treatment. This allows the patient to focus on the physical condition, which is your responsibility. When Roy Jones asked Mr. Phillips about his head, he built a bridge that supported their therapeutic intervention.

Once intervention begins, stay with the patient at all times. Erratic changes in behavior make it imperative to stay close to him. Your presence does more than just babysit the patient. You cannot only assess his level of consciousness, but you can also help to orient him by repeating your name, where you are, and your plan of intervention. Keep reminding him of these basic facts.

Attend

Intoxicated patients or patients in withdrawal may reveal a lot of deeply buried material. Even if some of the revelations seem unremarkable to you, they may reflect "dark secrets." Do not make light of or mock anything that you are told. As with overtly psychotic patients, do not buy into any stories that you do not believe, but do not belittle the storyteller either.

Document

As with any patient contact, it is important to document the patient's condition and your intervention. Physical findings must be fully documented—especially if the patient refuses further treatment. Homicidal or suicidal thoughts can be important considerations in later treatment. Quotes can be important. Under no circumstances should you write disparaging or derogatory remarks about the patient. Report physical observations about alcohol use objectively. Note the patient's motor control, level of consciousness, and so on. Resist the urge to describe the patient as a "town drunk" or "derelict." Finally, your careful documentation will support your claims that adequate care was rendered should this ever become an issue in a civil case.

 CONSIDERATIONS FOR EMS PROVIDERS

There are four important points to remember. First, addiction is a disease. It is not a matter of weak will. In fact, it has been rightly said that no one has a stronger will than the alcoholic seeking the next drink. Some EMS providers become hard-hearted toward addicts. They see the failures of the treatment system. They see the derelict who returns to the same street corner and sleeps in his own feces. They see the drunk driver who crashes himself and his passenger into a tree. They do not see the treatment successes. In fact, early intervention produces very high recovery rates. Alcoholics Anonymous is a worldwide fellowship of recovering alcoholics who testify convincingly to the ability of many people to recover.

Second, the drug scene is constantly changing. There are old standbys—alcohol, sleeping pills, amphetamines, cocaine and crack cocaine—but drug takers find unusual combinations and new ways to take drugs. Designer drugs alone and in combination create new problems in assessment and treatment.[15] EMS providers need to know what drugs are current on the streets of their communities. Any attempt to provide a list would surely be out of date by the time this book is published.

Third, it is important to recognize and deal with negative attitudes toward certain types of patients. This is important not only for patient care but because repeated, unsatisfactory encounters can lead to burnout. Perhaps one of the best ways to gain some perspective is to attend an open Alcoholics Anonymous meeting. At an open meeting anyone is welcome. Alcoholics Anonymous, listed in the telephone directory, can give you the time and location of an open meeting near you. Make sure you attend an open, not a closed meeting.

Fourth, EMS providers do become addicted themselves.[16,17] It is important to know the facts and the possibilities for dealing with addiction. Employee assistance programs (EAPs) can provide valuable help for a troubled helper.[18,19]

CONCLUSION

Alcohol abuse figures into a significant number of EMS responses. In some cases, it is a contributing factor—as in an early morning motor vehicle crash. In others, it is a direct cause—as in polydrug overdose. Still, in other cases, it is the underlying condition that brings a person to the attention of authorities—as in some "man down" calls. Your task is to appreciate the power of alcohol and treat the person with an alcohol problem as a person.

REVIEW QUESTIONS

1. Why might a person who abuses alcohol be unaware of the effects his or her behavior is having on others?
2. What is codependence? How might a codependent family member affect an alcoholic's treatment situation?
3. How might alcohol-abusing patients become involved with the EMS system?
4. How can an EMS provider approach an alcoholic to reduce his or her defensiveness?

EXERCISES

1. Attend an open Alcoholics Anonymous or Narcotics Anonymous meeting. Such an experience is amazing for many.
2. Find and then discuss the 12-Step Alcoholics Anonymous program.
3. Have a recovering person with a substance-abuse problem address your group.
4. Discuss the ways an EMS provider's personal experiences can shape reactions to alcoholics.

REFERENCES

1. Guttenberg, M., & Asaeda, G. (2002). Under the influence. *Journal of Emergency Medical Services, 27* (8), 50–52, 54–56, 58.
2. National Highway Traffic Safety Administration. (1989). Alcohol prevention curriculum for EMS providers. (DOT HS 900 093 NTS-42 3/89), p. 8.
3. Isselbacher, K. J. et al. (Eds.). (1980). *Harrison's principles of internal medicine,* (9th ed.). New York: McGraw-Hill.
4. Royce, J. (1981). *Alcohol problems and alcoholism.* New York: John Wiley & Sons.
5. Limmer, D. (2002). 10 commandments of EMS survival. *Journal of Emergency Medical Services, 25* (8), 24–30.
6. Beattie, M. (1996). *Codependent no more* (2nd ed.). New York: Hazeldon Information Education.
7. U.S. Department of Health, Education and Welfare. (1990). Alcohol and the central nervous system. In D. Ward (Ed.). *Alcoholism: introduction to theory and treatment* (3rd ed.) (pp. 39–40). Dubuque, IA: Kendall/Hunt.
8. U.S. Department of Health, Education and Welfare. (1990). Alcohol related illnesses. In D. Ward (Ed.). *Alcoholism: introduction to theory and treatment* (3rd ed.) (p. 59). Dubuque, IA: Kendall/Hunt.
9. Zinberg, N. (1981). Alcohol addiction: toward a more comprehensive definition. In M. Bean and N. Zinberg (Eds.). *Dynamic approaches to the understanding and treatment of alcoholism* (p. 97). New York: Free Press.
10. Galanter, M., & Kleber, H. D. (1999). *Textbook of substance abuse treatment* (2nd ed.). Washington, DC: American Psychiatric Press.
11. Goodwin, D. (1990). Alcohol problems in adoptees raised apart from alcoholic biological parents. In D. Ward (Ed.). *Alcoholism: introduction to theory and treatment* (3rd ed.) (p. 140). Dubuque, IA: Kendall/Hunt.

12. Seixa, J. S., & Geraldine, Y. (1985). *Children of alcoholism.* New York: Harper & Row.

13. Soreff, S. (2002). Suicide. *www.emedicine.com.*

14. Weissberg, M. (1983). *Dangerous secrets: maladaptive responses to stress.* New York: W. W. Norton.

15. Dillman, J. (1988). Designer drugs. *Journal of Emergency Medical Services, 13* (44), 44–47.

16. Maggiore, W. A. (1996). Substance abuse. *Journal of Emergency Medical Services, 21* (11), 66–67, 69, 71–72, 76–78, 80.

17. Avis, H. (1999). *Drugs and life* (4th ed.). New York: McGraw-Hill.

18. Howell, V. (1988). Taking care of the caretaker. *Journal of Emergency Medical Services, 13* (11), 38–45.

19. Mitchell, J., Bray, G. P., Mitchell, J. T. (1989). *Emergency Services Stress: Guidelines on Preserving the Health and Careers of Emergency Services Personnel,* Englewood Cliffs, NJ, Prentice-Hall.

FURTHER INFORMATION

Internet Resources

National Council on Alcoholism and Drug Dependence: www.ncadd.org

American Academy of Addiction Psychiatry: www.aaap.org

Media Resources

Movies

28 Days

Days of Wine and Roses

Leaving Las Vegas

Pulp Fiction

The Man with the Golden Arm

Train Spotting

When a Man Loves a Woman

Books

Any of Alcoholics Anonymous publications, for example, *One day at a time in al-anon.*

Miller, N. S. (1997). *The principles and practice of addictions in psychiatry.* Philadelphia: W. B. Saunders.

CHAPTER 11

The Unwanted

Deinstitutionalization, Detoxification, and Dereliction of Duty

 OBJECTIVES

Upon completion of this chapter, you should be able to:

- Describe the significance of homelessness in society and in your work.
- Describe the difficulties of assessing the homeless patient.
- Suggest ways to counteract negative feelings toward homeless patients.
- Identify ways that you can show concern rather than rejection.

THE CHALLENGE

There may be as many as 2 million homeless people in the United States for some period of time during a year. For some, homelessness is a temporary state. For others, it is a chronic condition.[1]

When we think of homeless people, we generally think of the resourceless people who dwell in the streets and shelters and single-room occupancy dwellings of large cities. Although in this chapter we focus on the urban homeless, we believe our comments apply more generally to people who might be labeled "The Unwanted." These unwanted people include residents of suburbs who must choose between paying for their shelter and meeting other needs such as food or heat, and also includes the rural poor who live in drafty shacks with inadequate facilities.

Many are middle-aged or elderly, some are young adults, some are families, and some are children without families. They have few champions, few strong alliances, and few drives—except the drive to survive from day to day, week to week, and season to season. The more we learn about them, the less we know. We stereotype them as addicted, mentally ill, or antisocial and avoid eye contact with "the homeless." Yet, beneath the surface similarities, the homeless are a highly diverse group of individuals, each with individual medical needs and a unique personal and medical history. In fact, the fastest growing group are families with children. These homeless are often invisible because they do not fit our stereotypes.[1] The challenge for the EMS provider is to maintain professional objectivity, to assist in the caring process, and to intervene at the level required. The EMS provider's job is complicated by the fact that the EMS system is often the only route into the health care system for a homeless individual. Frequently, it is the only ongoing support for this population. The professional challenge is first and foremost to recognize that an individual who is homeless is not personless.

E. Fuller Torrey suggests the situation is a national disgrace characterized by inadequate and inept social policies.[2] EMS is forced into the front lines in the care for the homeless, and EMS providers are left to deal with the human consequences of social failure.

 THE PATIENT AND THE SITUATION

Looking older than his 41 years, short, squat Sheldon "Shelly" Fairlawn ambles through the entranceway of the counter service section of Ralph's Diner. It is 10:00 A.M. The breakfast crowd has gone, and there are a few solitary men and women scattered throughout the quick meal section. The manager sometimes lets Shelly sit with a cup of coffee if he comes between the breakfast and lunch hours.

Shelly has a distinctive, hacking cough. In a coughing fit, he becomes unsteady on his feet and leans for support on a trash container. He does not grip it firmly enough and crumbles to the ground. The manager had seen him come in, heard his noisy cough, and was on his way to escort him out of the restaurant. The manager finds Shelly lying on his side on the floor, one hand on his chest, coughing noisily. Shelly is bothered by the scene he is causing and very concerned that he has injured his leg. He has been living with two other men in an abandoned building and has not gone to the homeless shelter since one of the other residents attacked him for his shoes about 3 weeks ago.

He has moved between residence hotels, the shelter, and the streets for several months, but he has not adjusted to homelessness. He had a job at the Jupiter Supermarket last year but lost it when the chain went into Chapter 11 bankruptcy. They eliminated many positions, including Shelly's graveyard shift job restocking shelves. He did his job, never missed work, and followed simple orders to the letter. He had no close friends and did not want any. He lost contact with his family several months after he lost his job.

Two things stand out about Shelly on this day, and neither has any direct relationship to his injury. The first is his attire; the second is his odor. He is disheveled, dirty, and smelly. His jacket is too large, but in another sense too

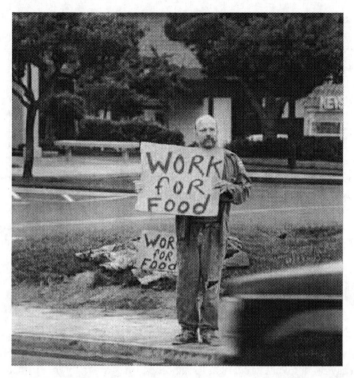

(Courtesy of Morton Beebe-S.F./Corbis)

small—it fails to keep him warm in the bitter cold of this seaport city in mid-February. His pants are worn and discolored. The left knee has a large "smile" on it. His bright lime green socks match nothing else in his wardrobe and draw attention to his boat shoes. The lime socks provide a beacon in a foggy seascape. His shirt comes from Brooks Brothers by way of Goodwill Industries. Perhaps the most striking thing about Shelly, however, is his smell. It is a strong, repulsive odor of which Shelly is completely unaware. It is a result of Shelly's infrequent washing, compounded by his living in smoke- and alcohol-filled rooms. In part it is a smell that attached itself to Shelly's clothes before he ever wore them.

A small group gathers around, but not close to, Mr. Fairlawn. They are more curious than caring. The manager focuses his efforts on getting him out of the restaurant. He asks him if he is all right. Shelly says—somewhat unclearly—that he hurts and does not think he can move. The manager urges him to give it a try, though he does not physically help him. The manager asks his assistant to call 911. He reports to the dispatcher only that a customer has fallen, may have injured his back and leg, and is in a great deal of pain. The assistant does not describe Mr. Fairlawn's other conditions. After all, they don't want the ambulance crew to hold back because Mr. Fairlawn is "just a bum."

Paul and Sam proceed to Ralph's Diner. As they enter, they experience a sense of déjà vu. From across the room, they recognize Shelly's lime green socks. Shelly's socks are well known. He finds—heaven knows how—the gaudiest colors imaginable. His one concession to proper dress is that they are always the same color.

Paul feels momentarily embarrassed when he sees "old lime socks." Paul and Sam move quickly down the aisle. They introduce themselves to Mr. Fairlawn, and Paul asks, "What hurts?"

The examination yields evidence of ankle injury. At first Mr. Fairlawn balks at the idea of going to the emergency department (ED), wondering how he can possibly get back to his "apartment." Sam assures him that Jack Morton, the social worker at the ED, will help him somehow.

En route, Paul rides in back with Shelly. Shelly tells him about how he lost his job at Jupiter. Paul, it turns out, has a cousin who also lost a job there. Paul and Shelly complain about the economy and the hypocrisy of city hall.

 ## THE PATIENT'S WORLD

Street people are a mystery to almost everyone who works a regular job and returns to a fixed residence at night. To some they are "poor unfortunates," who should be locked up for their own good. To others they are harmless buffoons who really do not want to change. To still others, they are frightening lunatics capable of thoughtless violence. In fact, they are a diverse group with very different needs and problems.[3] All definitions are inadequate, but, however defined, they share homelessness and a lack of connectedness to other people.

Homelessness represents an underlying common denominator, but the reasons why the homeless have no place to live are diverse. Drug or alcohol use may be a factor, but many alcoholics and drug addicts are not homeless. Social rejection may be a factor, but many people who are rejected by their families still manage to hold on to a residence and a job. Mental illness may be a factor, but many people who are mentally ill manage to live in sheltered settings. In the final analysis, each street person has a unique story to tell. For Shelly, he has reached the streets through an isolated life-style, a bankruptcy, and difficulty in bouncing back.

The homeless survive economically by restricting their needs. Some do temporary jobs requiring little skill and little contact with the public; some collect returnable bottles; some beg for money on a corner or inside a doorway; some sell small quantities of drugs; some wipe the windshields of cars stopped at traffic lights; some sell their bodies. Some hang out in parks, some in public libraries, still others in shelters.

What is constant is that the vast majority of their activities are concerned with immediate survival. Few have more resources than they need to get through a day or a week. Shelly had been trained and was comfortable in his job. He finds work other than night shift work too stressful. If he cannot find night work, the insecurities of the streets are less threatening than the insecurities of a day job around other people. Of course, his lifestyle becomes a vicious cycle: a person who is unkempt at an interview is unlikely to be hired, a person without a fixed address cannot receive job applications or acceptances, and prospective employers are less than enthusiastic about hiring a person who lists a hotel or a shelter as an address.

Many chronic forms of mental illness as well as severe acute episodes contribute to the inability to maintain a home or a job. Up to one-third of street dwellers have a previous psychiatric history. Several consequences of severe illness predispose individuals to homelessness: inability to concentrate, inability to stay in one geographic location for an extended time, problems of controlling thoughts or the intrusion of delusions or hallucinations, deficiencies in interpersonal skills, and a lack of basic abilities. Coupled with all this is a significant bias against hiring the mentally ill. Deinstitutionalization from mental hospitals was supposed to return the patient to the community. Too often it returns them to the streets.

Public hospitals are becoming the primary health-care providers for the uninsured poor. Small rural hospitals find their resources similarly stressed. Their main routes into those facilities are on foot or by ambulance. The homeless do need health services. Many needs arise directly from their living conditions. Obviously, there are exposure-related conditions, respiratory diseases, infestations, injuries, and psychological problems.

 ## THE BEHAVIOR OF THE PATIENT

Homeless behavior runs toward extremes. Many of the homeless are deeply subservient and docile. Others are agitated and act out when forced to interact. Either situation complicates assessment and care. For some, the streets represent a way in which they can live an "uninvolved" life. The ability to adopt this personal style may be a consequence of remote parenting that they received, being hurt in relationships too many times, or one extremely painful hurt. Some people see relationships as a burden that they do not desire. For some, substance abuse—especially alcoholism—becomes a way of life that precludes closeness. The ability to get the next drink becomes life's sole focus and purpose.

 ## THE EMOTIONS AND THOUGHTS BEHIND THE BEHAVIOR

Often, the emotional life of the homeless is restricted. For some it is restricted by the need to invest energy in getting from one end of the day to the other. For others, it is characterized by sadness born of chronic losses or by a **flat affect** such as is seen in schizophrenic disorders or organic mental disorders (often seen in patients with dementia or chronic alcoholism). Others may appear disoriented or incredibly unconcerned about their environment due to head trauma or to chronic drug use.

No one thought pattern characterizes the homeless. Some show signs of a thought disorder such as schizophrenia—speaking in loose associations that are hard to follow. Some show **thought blocking**, experience hallucinations and delusions, or have a sense that others are controlling their thoughts. Others may be focused on the next bottle or the next hit.

 ## FAMILY/BYSTANDER RESPONSES

The homeless call out a surprising range of reactions. Bystander responses will range from pity and concern to scorn and repulsion. Any one of these reactions can motivate bystanders to call for help when they see a homeless man or woman sleeping or passed out in a public place or on steps. Some bystanders will feel "There, but for the grace of God, go I"; others may want to see the authorities remove a blight on the neighborhood.

A bystander who is concerned that a homeless person be treated with dignity and respect may watch EMS providers as closely as if the EMS providers were caring for a member of his or her own family. At the other extreme, a store manager who is concerned with negative attention that might be drawn to a business may wish that the person be removed as quickly as possible and may be impatient with assessment and spinal immobilization.

 ## PROVIDER RESPONSES

Treating the deinstitutionalized mental patient or the alcoholic derelict who makes his or her home in various shelters can be a frustrating experience. EMS providers may see any intervention as futile. They may even think that death is a blessed relief for "those people." The experienced urban EMS provider has seen "one-legged Melvin," or "Frankie" or "Sophie" on the street for years. The partners of new EMS providers point out the bottle gang that hangs on the corner in the first few trips through the neighborhood and tell stories of past encounters. They joke that, "When we pick up Frankie, he's out of the ED before we are." The "alkies" or the "weirdos" with a tendency to get nasty or spit are singled out for special attention.

Working with the homeless can spill over into home life as well. A worker who's been around a homeless man or woman picks up a certain odor, which he can unwittingly take home with him. This situation can be dealt with easily. It is more difficult when the contact begins to breed contempt either for homeless people or for the system that allows them to live that way.

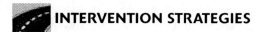 **INTERVENTION STRATEGIES**

Observe

In contrast to the other patients we have described, or will describe, the homeless patient's clothing is probably more important than his setting. Clothing, especially in relationship to weather, can give you three important clues.

First, a man who is obviously underdressed on a cold day may be a candidate for hypothermia—especially if he has been drinking. A man who is overdressed on a warm day may show signs of heat exhaustion.

Second, the general state of a person's clothing will tell you much about his or her self-image. Many "bag ladies" make a point of only dressing in clean, once fashionable clothes. The clothes may be obvious discards, but they are of high quality. At the extreme is the person who puts together a wardrobe out of any combination.

Third, grass stains, dirt, or particles of twig or brush on clothing will suggest a person who has been sleeping outdoors, rather than in a shelter. This, of course, is not hard and fast, but a shelter resident is more likely to receive medical attention.

A careful assessment is important. Skin condition will reveal signs of dehydration (tenting), cyanosis, or liver disease (jaundice). Other conditions can also be identified from skin appearance. Obscene or vulgar tattoos may suggest a person with a tendency toward aggression or antisocial behavior. Slash marks on wrists or rope burns on neck may suggest suicidal tendencies. "Tracks" suggest IV drug use.

However, the setting can be important. Note personal belongings that might be carried in a shopping cart or in bags. Pay attention to the person's living condition, which may be relevant to posthospitalization placement.

Interact

For the reasons identified previously—communication difficulties, drug use, inadequate personality—you may have to depend more on signs than symptoms in assessing the patient. Do not assume that the patient cannot participate in treatment. Different parts of a city attract different types of street people. A homeless man in a fast-food restaurant is likely to be considerably more comfortable in interaction than one found "in the weeds." Treat the man or woman with respect. Pet nicknames or terms such as "dearie" or "buddy" are not appropriate. Unless proven otherwise, assume that he or she can participate in care decisions. There are good reasons for not shrinking from interaction. Professionally, you have an obligation to respond without prejudice. Further, a respectful approach reduces the likelihood that the patient will act out. People take their cues from many different sources. The less you appear like "the law" and more like a helper, the less threatening you appear. In general, detoxification center workers and shelter workers experience few problems with acting out behavior.

A different case for treatment without prejudice is illustrated in the following story told by James Page. An illegal alien, a derelict alcoholic, was struck on the head by an unknown assailant and left in the street. The EMS providers who came on the call left him at the scene. He died of an undiagnosed subdural hematoma. The man had a son who had a lawyer. "The paramedics had called the drunken, dirty patient, 'an old puke.' The son and the lawyer showed the paramedics and their employer that an 'old puke' is worth $300,000 in that town."[4]

Ask

Do not assume that there is nothing wrong with a homeless "man down." Asking what seems to be the trouble will cue you in to the person's general level of orientation. Many homeless people are well-oriented to person, place, and time. Inquiring about past treatments, including medical and psychiatric hospitalizations, will help identify the presence of chronic disease or psychosis. A medical history should include information on drugs taken (or not taken) recently. Since tuberculosis (TB) is common in some homeless populations, check for a positive history or for prescribed TB medications. Current or recent alcohol use is important. Rather than assuming alcoholism, find out about current drinking. An alcoholic who has not been drinking recently may go into withdrawal.

Act

As with any patient, standard precautions are appropriate. In addition, if the patient's body odor is interfering with your objectivity, you may find it helpful, as one EMS provider suggested, to place a small dab of a medicated ointment such as Vapo-Rub under your nose.

Be careful in removing any of the patient's clothing. Some homeless alcoholics will have leg ulcers or sores or may have open cuts that will have bled against clothing.

Attend

As with any other patient, do not leave the patient alone. Your continued presence prevents further injury and conveys the message of care and hope. Listen to what the patient might have to say, but do not support any fantastic or ridiculous claims that he or she might make. Do not abandon the patient. Be certain that if the patient refuses treatment or transport, it is his or her wish, not yours.

Document

Document the encounter with a homeless person as you would any encounter. Do not write derogatory remarks on the run report. Describing a person as a "town drunk" or an "old puke" is clearly unprofessional. Likewise, if a person has no fixed address, do not write "the weeds," on the address line, as funny as it might seem at the time.

CONSIDERATIONS FOR EMS PROVIDERS

The homeless population poses a special challenge. You may be their primary health-care provider. Some EMS providers will sense a tremendous injustice in the social system. Some will feel outrage at being placed in this position. Regardless of your feelings, remember that you are often a lifeline. The more you learn about the homeless, the more their individual characteristics emerge. The more you can respond to the patient as an individual, the less resentment you will feel and the better the job you will do.

If you work with a service that transports homeless individuals on a regular basis, you should consider meeting with shelter workers and public detoxification center workers to learn more about specific problems and solutions. On the job, you cannot solve society's problems. Off duty, if you want to do something about the problem of homelessness, there are many ways to become involved, from donating time to the construction of affordable housing units to volunteering with a shelter program.

CONCLUSION

Homelessness is not just an urban problem; it is found in suburbs and rural areas as well. It may not be as obvious in the countryside as in a major city. In some areas, the unwanted may not actually be "homeless"—they may have inadequate homes: drafty shacks, overcrowded, illegally occupied dwellings. These are people who are stigmatized; their needs are complicated by rejection. This rejection complicates the work of those on the frontlines of human services. It will lead many homeless to delay care until they can only be helped through the EMS system. It will lead some citizens to use public services in "cleaning up the neighborhood." The communication challenges can be great—as in working with substance-abusing patients and with confrontational patients. It may be difficult, but it is important to remember that your primary mission is to provide care to the best of your ability.

REVIEW QUESTIONS

1. What are three conditions that might lead to a person becoming homeless?

2. What types of medical needs would you expect to find in the homeless population?

3. What are some of the communications difficulties you might experience in working with a homeless person?

EXERCISES

1. Serve a meal at a homeless shelter. The more you know about the homeless the easier it is to provide adequate, unbiased care.
2. Visit a state hospital.
3. Have a homeless person address your group.
4. Do homeless persons choose their lifestyle? Discuss this subject with your group.

REFERENCES

1. nwrel.org/cfc/fre/pdf/Handout2.pdf.
2. Torry, E. F. (1988). *Nowhere to go.* New York: Harper & Row, p. 199.
3. http://aspe.os.dhhs.gov/progsys/homeless/2002
4. Page, J. O. (1988). Perspective on prejudice. *Journal of Emergency Medical Services, 13* (4), p. 5.

FURTHER INFORMATION

Internet Resources

National Law Center on Homelessness and Poverty: www.nlchp.org

Federal government information on homelessness: http://aspe.os. dhhs.gov/progsys/homeless/

U.S. Department of Housing and Urban Development: www.hud.gov/ homeless.html

Media Resources

Movies
Grapes of Wrath

The Fisher King

Books
Cobb, J. (Ed.). (1999). *The way home: ending homelessness in America.* New York: Harry N. Abrams.

Kusmer, K. L. (2001). *Down & out, on the road: the homeless in American history.* New York: Oxford University Press.

CHAPTER 12

Provocative Patients

The Sexy, the Suit Conscious, and the Somatizing

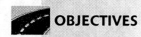 **OBJECTIVES**

Upon completion of this chapter, you should be able to:

- Recognize how we all try to present an idealized self on occasion.
- Recognize that for some patients, creating or maintaining a particular role may be more important than providing direct answers to your assessment questions
- Recognize that there is a crucial difference between putting a patient at ease and becoming involved in a fantasy.
- Recognize that a patient who is contemplating a lawsuit may want to involve you in matters that exceed your emergency medical competence.
- Recognize that a patient who is overly concerned with medical conditions may provide misleading or inaccurate but very plausible information.
- Explain how documentation is important in each of these situations.

THE CHALLENGE

Not all the challenges in emergency care come from working in difficult environments and making complicated assessment and emergency care decisions. Some come from patients with complicated psychological needs. This chapter presents three scenarios: the seductive patient, the **litigious** patient, and the **somatizing,** or hypochondriacal, patient. These cases are representative of some of the most frequently encountered provocative patients. In our scenarios, the patients' physical conditions are uncomplicated, but the conditions that the patients' personalities impose on the EMS providers are complicated indeed.

The challenge is to focus on the immediate treatment needs of your patient and your ability to meet those needs within your scope of training. Doing this, you not only serve these patients but improve your service to all your patients. The proper methods for caring for provocative patients are, generally, appropriate methods for use in caring for all patients.

THE SEDUCTIVE PATIENT

 THE PATIENT AND THE SITUATION

During the lunch hour crush, 22-year-old Brenda Harewood slips and falls on a plastic shirt bag in Murdoch's Department Store. She was passing through the men's section on her way to misses' casual wear. She is wearing a short, tight skirt—a skirt that tests the limits of her employer's dress code—and a floral print blouse. She falls solidly on her left thigh. A security guard and a clerk, both of whom were watching her entrance, rush to her aid.

Brenda lies in the middle of the aisle. A small group congregates about her. "I feel numb," she says. "I can't move my leg." A middle-aged man sternly commands, "Don't move. Stay still. Don't move anything." Another man volunteers to get help.

Brenda does not try to move. A small group of men—sales clerks and customers—has gathered. The department manager comes over and asks what has happened. One of the clerks explains, "This young lady fell in the aisle." Brenda points toward the shiny, plastic wrapper beside her thigh.

In response to the 911 call, EMS providers Paul Appleton and Sam Peppers arrive within 3 minutes. A security guard points them in Brenda's direction. Paul, perhaps unconsciously, stands taller and becomes more aggressive in ordering shoppers out of his way when he sees Brenda. Paul seems to be enjoying the role of rescuer. Sam, with his greater experience, intuitively feels that Paul could make a fool of himself. As they approach, they notice that the top three buttons of Brenda's blouse are open.

Paul introduces himself and Sam. Brenda introduces herself in turn. Paul asks, "What seems to be wrong?" Brenda explains that she slipped on the plastic shirt wrapper. "Someone told me not to move, so I just stayed where I fell."

Paul assures her that she did the right thing. She tells the EMS providers that her left leg feels numb. Her thigh is beginning to hurt. Sam explains, "I'm going to hold your neck and head still. Just in case you have some other injuries, we wouldn't want you to make them worse by moving." Paul explains that before they begin any treatment they are going to have to check for other injuries.

Brenda asks, with a slight smile on her face, "Am I going to like this?" Before he can answer, Brenda reaches out and clasps Paul's hand. "I'm so glad you're here." Perhaps her statement is an innocent expression of gratitude. Perhaps

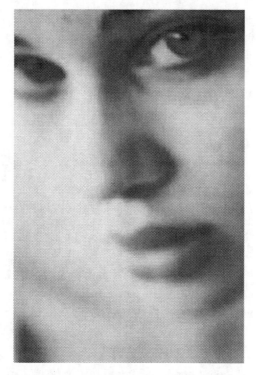

(Courtesy of EyeWire)

it is a lead into a less innocent conversation. She certainly makes Paul feel needed. It is a satisfying feeling.

Paul pulls out his latex gloves. As he starts to put them on, Brenda says, "I believe in safe sex, but you really don't take any chances." She adds, "You won't catch anything from me. I hope I couldn't catch anything from you."

Sam clears his throat, breaking into this conversation. "Ms. Harewood, these are standard procedures we take with every patient." Paul feels gently behind her neck and over her shoulders. Brenda looks intently into his eyes. Paul moves his hands down her sides pressing her ribs gently. She stiffens visibly at his touch but says casually in a soft voice "Do you like what you feel?" Paul says, "You're in great shape." Brenda says, "Well, knowing I'm in good hands makes me feel better." Sam breaks in, "My partner is checking to make sure that you don't have any obvious injuries to your ribs. He'll check your back and pelvis next." Paul, responding to Sam's tone, adopts a more professional stance. Before he continues his assessment, he calmly asks the crowd to stand back. He tells Brenda that, as much as he likes to joke around sometimes, some of the people there might "get the wrong idea." Brenda smiles coyly and says, "You're the doctor.

I'm in your hands." Paul doubts that Brenda really understands that he should not be joking with her. But he and Sam complete their assessment, treatment, and transport without incident.

 ## THE PATIENT'S WORLD

A seductive patient often presents a series of contradictions. The patient's dress and language suggest a degree of familiarity and comfort with sexual experience. The patient may flirt or engage in witty banter in public. However, body language and facial expression may show doubt or reserve. Often, serious internal struggles with body identity and sexuality are only vaguely—if at all—recognized by the patient. The same person who seems poised and confident in public may be aloof and anxious in a situation in which intimate sexual contact is a possibility.

Our example involves a woman, but men can also be seductive. A seductive male patient can similarly challenge the professionalism of female EMS providers.

 ## THE BEHAVIOR OF THE PATIENT

The hallmark of the seductive patient's behavior is provocative activity—verbal and physical—designed to sexually attract another person. In many settings puns, jokes with a sexual theme, and light banter is welcome and appropriate among friends. In the context of a medical emergency, such behavior is clearly inappropriate. For the EMS provider, bantering in response is also inappropriate.

Verbal behaviors range from seemingly lighthearted inquiry into the EMS provider's private life to inappropriate, intimate revelations. At one extreme, it may be as simple as the question, "Are you doing anything after work tonight?" At the other extreme, it may range to unsolicited, needless comments on erogenous zones. "Men usually only touch me there with the lights out."

Physical behaviors center around display or a lack of modesty. A low-cut dress or unbuttoned blouse may be perfectly appropriate in some settings, and standards of modesty differ, but a seductive display is marked by (1) exaggerated posing that emphasizes the body parts in question and (2) affectionate touching not warranted by the situation. Brenda may not be aware that her dress style differs sharply from that of the other women in the office.

 ## THE EMOTIONS AND THOUGHTS BEHIND THE BEHAVIOR

Sexually provocative patients may not be conscious of their provocation, or they may consciously push themselves toward the helper. For example, a woman who "likes a man in uniform" may be very forward, emphasizing how much she is drawn to the uniform. At the other extreme, a woman may be extremely naive, with little insight into the effect she is producing.

The causes of sexually provocative behavior are varied. For some, arousing another sexually draws attention away from one's inadequacies; for others, it is a way of avoiding emotional intimacy. Actually giving sexual favors, however, is condemned by family, church, and peers. In essence, thoughts and feelings run in the opposite direction from outward behavior. Some male patients will display biceps to gain attention and recognition. This behavior may be a compensation for inadequacy in other realms.

In other cases, there may be a definite psychopathology involved. These cases may involve a **regression,** or return to an immature level of functioning in the face of overwhelming stress. in other words, under stress, the patient reverts to a less developed form of behavior. He or she exhibits openness and dependency and wants to be cared for.

In neither type of situation is the EMS provider the actual stimulus for the sexual display, and despite the provocative behavior, the EMS provider should not respond in kind.

 ## BYSTANDER RESPONSES

An attractive patient may draw substantial attention, and an openly seductive one may seem to crave such attention. While most patients who are injured in public desire privacy, a seductive patient, like the other patient types described in this chapter, may seek attention for his or her own needs.

 ## PROVIDER RESPONSES

A provocative patient can elicit two very strong but very different types of reactions. The first is attraction or interest. The other is disdain. In our scenario, Paul Appleton finds himself literally racing down the aisle to help Brenda. The situation fits his fantasy of being a rescuer. The danger—and it is probably greater for a male EMS provider and a female patient than for a female EMS provider and a male patient—is that the EMS provider is drawn into the patient's world instead of drawing the patient into the world of treatment. Paul must ask Brenda for her address and phone number for documentation purposes, but he must not ask what she's doing that night, even as a joke. He must not tell too much about his personal situation. The fact that he is divorced or "available" is not relevant to Brenda's care.

Disdain follows from an entirely different reading of the situation. It may relate to a "once bitten, twice shy," reaction. The disdainful EMS provider may have seen other EMS providers make fools of themselves, or worse, and may associate Brenda's behavior with promiscuity or otherwise value it negatively.

Neither approach is correct. To the extent that the patient's behavior is controlling the EMS provider, it is undercutting the treatment relationship.

 INTERVENTION STRATEGIES

Observe

The most important point to be made about observation is not to be distracted by the obvious. If the patient is attractive, his or her appearance may draw your attention away from other features of the environment.

Interact

Address the patient formally, for example, "Ms. Harewood," unless given permission to do otherwise. If the patient requests that you use a first name, do so in a matter-of-fact manner. Do not suggest any special familiarity in the way you address the patient. It is essential not to be distracted by the patient's display or banter. The best advice is to follow a course of interaction that would be equally appropriate with an older woman or with a man in the same situation. As appropriate, ask permission to touch the patient and explain what you are doing.

Ask

You must ask only pertinent questions. Never suggest that you have a personal interest in any answer. For example, you need an emergency contact for your records, but it is irrelevant to you personally if the patient is married.

Act

Stay in control of the situation. Do not let the patient define the conditions under which you work.

Attend

Listen carefully to what the patient says, but do not necessarily believe it. Many of the things a seductive patient will say are flattering. Flattery is, by definition, a compliment given to further the objectives of the speaker.

Document

Record meaningful patient care information. Avoid comments about dress or behavior.

THE LITIGIOUS PATIENT

 THE PATIENT AND THE SITUATION

During the lunch hour crush, 42-year-old Gordon Hale slips and falls on a plastic shirt bag in Murdoch's Department Store. He was picking through men's

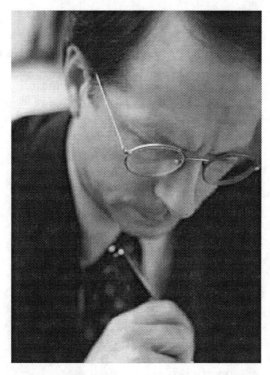

(Courtesy of PhotoDisc)

shirts looking for a plain white shirt in his size. He is dressed conservatively—dark blue suit, tie, white shirt, over-the-calf socks, and wing tips. He falls sideways, landing sharply on his left thigh. His left arm breaks his fall.

A security guard and a clerk, hearing the thud, rush to see what has happened. The security guard starts to help Gordon to his feet. A middle-aged man says, "Don't move him, he could have hurt his spine. Stay still. Don't move anything." Another says, "I'll get help." Although he does not seem in any acute distress, Gordon does not try to move. Apart from a pain in his wrist, where he landed, and a pain in his left thigh and buttocks, he felt nothing. Now he begins to wonder about a numbness in his leg. The department manager comes over and asks what has happened. One of the clerks explains, "This man fell in the aisle. We don't think we should move him until the ambulance arrives."

Gordon now seriously doubts that he can walk. In fact, he feels his other leg becoming numb. The assembled crowd looks on with a concern that he begins to reflect. The manager, following protocol, reports the incident to the chief of security.

Mr. Hale pulls a small black notebook out of his suitcoat pocket. He quickly notes the time of day and aisle location and asks the bystanders if they saw what happened. No one observed the fall, but several agree that it was just terrible for the store to let those things lie around. He gets names and addresses from two men.

Alice Turner, the security director, greets Mr. Hale cordially. She notes his obvious concern and his notebook. Mr. Hale asks, "Who are you? What is your position here?" She takes a deep breath, pauses, ignores the evident hostility, and answers his question. "Did you call a doctor or an ambulance?" Ms. Turner assures him that an ambulance has been called. Ms. Turner's presence actually serves two functions. One is to make sure that no further harm comes to the victim. The other is to make sure that none of her staff makes statements that could be used against Murdoch's.

In response to the 911 call, Paul Appleton and Sam Peppers arrive within 3 minutes. A security guard points them in Gordon's direction. Paul, perhaps unconsciously, relaxes and becomes less aggressive in ordering shoppers out of his way when he sees Mr. Hale. This patient fits Paul's stereotype of the patient with a minor sprain or strain. He guesses, correctly that Mr. Hale is writing in a notepad, recording the time the ambulance arrived and has taken down the name of the service from Paul's shoulder patch before they even introduce themselves. When they introduce themselves, Mr. Hale writes down their names and badge numbers.

"What seems to be wrong?"

Mr. Hale does not answer immediately. He asks petulantly, "What took you so long?" Paul Appleton is taken aback. He wants to make a rude comment, but he does not. Sam feels a catch in his throat and wonders about malpractice. Mr. Hale explains that he lost his footing on the plastic shirt wrapper that was left lying on the floor. He produces the wrapper in evidence. "Someone told me not to move, so I stayed right where I landed." He explains that his left leg feels numb. His thigh is beginning to hurt. He worries about possible wrist injury and—could it be possible?—a slipped disk.

Paul gently clears away the few hangers-on. He assures Mr. Hale that they will be checking him over and will be taking him to the hospital after they have taken care of any immediate problems that they find. Right now, just in case he has hurt his back, they want to put a collar on him and place him on a long board. Mr. Half realizes he will not be able to write any more. He puts down his notepad and asks, "Am I going to be all right?" Sam resists the temptation to offer easy reassurance. He says, "We'll do everything we can for you. I'll tell you what we find and what we are going to do as we treat you. If you have any questions, please ask." Mr. Hale repeats, in a public voice, most everything the EMS providers say to him. This repetition guarantees that he has witnesses to his version of events.

Sam follows his assessment protocols rigorously. Mr. Hale asks, "Do you see the goddamn bag these fools left lying around? That's what caused this mess." Sam answers, noncommittally, that he sees the bag on the floor. He avoids any light remarks that might suggest he is making fun of Mr. Hale. He also avoids casting any blame on the store. Mr. Hale also asks about the bill. This is not an unexpected question. Paul gives the standard answer, straight from the policy manual.

The assessment, spine boarding, and splinting proceed unremarkably. Before lifting Mr. Hale to the stretcher, Sam and Paul explain what they will do.

 ## THE PATIENT'S WORLD

A number of patients may take a litigious stance following an injury. The possibilities of compensation are tantalizing. Newspapers report jury awards of $500,000 or more for emotional damages. Some patients may be inclined to exact punishment from the guilty party because of a religious or philosophical orientation. Litigation is a possibility in almost any case. However, the litigious patient is one who takes a stance in which his interest in litigation may impede your ability to conduct an adequate assessment and treatment.

 ## THE BEHAVIOR OF THE PATIENT

The litigious patient insists on rights and is concerned that you explain what you are doing and that you follow those explanations precisely in providing care. Further, the litigious patient may attempt to document everything. One EMS provider reports that one evening when his crew went to transport a chronic obstructive pulmonary disease (COPD) patient, the patient's family videotaped everything they did. The litigious patient may try to direct and reorganize the situation in specific ways.

First, a litigious patient is typically knowledgeable of his or her rights and will assert these. For example, Mr. Hale demands of the director of security that a doctor or an ambulance be called. Even if the patient is factually wrong about what those rights are, he or she will assert these beliefs as gospel.

Second, such persons often demand adherence to procedure. Mr. Hale does not know the proper treatment for his condition, whatever that is, but he asks the EMS providers to verbalize what they will do, where they will take him, and how long it will take to get there. And, he makes sure that either their statements or his paraphrase of their statements are heard by witnesses.

Third, a litigation-minded patient is likely to write down every detail, even asking for the name of an EMS supervisor.

In fairness, it must be pointed out that these patients are not necessarily wrong. The injury may not be their fault, and they may, in fact, be able to recover damages. At issue is their behavior during the emergency response.

THE EMOTIONS AND THOUGHTS BEHIND THE BEHAVIOR

In the face of adversity, a litigious patient begins from a position that (1) he or she has been wronged; (2) someone must pay; and (3) the responsible person must be found. In contrast to the patient who is "out of control," this patient may appear to be in complete control of emotions and behaviors—calculating responses oriented toward establishing responsibility in addition to relieving pain. One of the hallmarks of this type of patient is that he or she tends to think rather than feel. The patient may not even know what his or her real feelings are.[1]

This patient feels angry and thinks he is entitled to some compensation for his suffering or embarrassment. Annoyance, righteous indignation, and discomfort are the most common emotional responses. These emotional responses are often conveyed through tone of voice and style of relating to others present. He may be excessively concerned with the question of who is to blame.

A patient may take a position for one or more of four different reasons. The patient himself may not even be conscious of the reasons for his behavior. Most important, his behavior is not simply a response to the EMS provider's treatment.

First, a patient's interest in solving problems through confrontation and litigation may go back to early life experiences. A family that emphasized injustice, conflict, and competition may instill such an attitude in children.

Second, this approach may be a defense against powerlessness. In a helping situation, the patient often feels helpless. This feeling can give rise to the very opposite need: the need for some control. The defiant stance will force caregivers (and others) to pay attention to the patient as a force, not just a body.

Third, some litigious patients respond out of hurt. They hurt so much that they want to ensure that someone will pay for it.

Fourth, there is the paranoid patient. For this patient, the world consists of enemies and ineffective allies. Enemies must be brought to justice.

Other patients may initiate lawsuits, but typically these patients will think about suing for justice, monetary gain, or revenge after the care has been delivered. The hallmark of a litigious patient is that he or she is already formulating a detailed case while you are providing care.

 ## BYSTANDER RESPONSES

A litigious patient may actually seek bystander support for his allegations. Before help has arrived on the scene, he may have actively involved bystanders in creating a legal case. Further, he may involve them in establishing a situation that presents the mechanism of injury as more serious than it was.

PROVIDER RESPONSES

The litigious patient can be extremely frustrating because he or she demands a great deal of information and asks questions that seem to question the abilities of the EMS providers. It is important to remember that this person's questions are not necessarily prompted by specific errors made by EMS providers, but are, rather, a way of approaching the world and handling anxiety. In the heat of the situation, it is difficult to remember that the confrontational behavior is not generated by the EMS providers or their treatment but has other sources.

EMS providers, nurses, and physicians are trained to help. A controlled— and controlling—patient such as Mr. Hale may engender discomfort and resentment. The health-care team may feel misunderstood. They may feel that they are becoming victims, with their professionalism and their jobs threatened. They feel that the manipulative information seeking is a personal attack. Their frustration may erupt into sarcasm or may result in lowered attention to the basics of care or lead to the practice of expensive "defensive medicine." Either result gives the litigious patient more to complain about.

INTERVENTION STRATEGIES

Observe

Your assessment of the scene should normally include an assessment of hazards and obstacles. The litigious patient is concerned with these hazards as well. It is important to remain independent and not to be unduly influenced by the patient's assessment of danger.

Interact

The key to dealing with a litigious patient is professionalism and teamwork. This should begin with introductions. Address the patient formally. Call him "Mr. Hale," not "Gordon" or "Gordee," unless he specifically indicates this is how he wishes to be addressed.

Small talk can ease the patient's mind in an unfamiliar situation. With a potentially litigious patient, it is important to avoid jokes that might be misinterpreted or cryptic remarks that might be considered hostile. Also avoid blaming or downgrading anyone else who might have offered to help. Do not withhold information.

In some situations, family members may be present. In these cases, the following rules apply. First, do not talk to the family without the patient's permission. Second, avoid offhand references about the patient's behavior. Do not make side comments such as "What's with the notepad?" or "I wonder if he's always this stiff?" If they are present, family members may feel the patient's behavior is totally appropriate. Third, keep your relationship professional. Do not joke or demean the patient or the situation. Know your billing practices. Provide accurate information.

Ask

This patient, like every other patient, is entitled to a thorough assessment. It is important to ask about and document the patient's chief complaint fully, to record any symptoms mentioned, and to take a thorough medical history. The questions that must be asked in developing a record of your care are the questions that must be asked in any thorough assessment.

Act

As with questioning, there are no special activities required. The greatest danger may be practicing what is sometimes called "**defensive medicine.**" Defensive medicine is overanalyzing, or overtreating, a patient because of the fear of a lawsuit.

Attend

A litigious patient may expect you to listen carefully. Your active listening may be very important to him or her. In fact, your listening may be taken as an indication of the quality of care you are providing. Eye contact is especially important.

Document

This record, more than others, may be likely to show up in a court action. Record neatly. Document all times, locations, and adherence to standards and protocols. A notation of mileage before leaving the scene and on arrival at the hospital, along with transport times will serve to document that you transported appropriately. Avoid judgments or comments that ascribe accusation and fault.

THE SOMATIZING PATIENT

 THE PATIENT AND THE SITUATION

During the lunch hour crush, 52-year-old Sarah Paine slips and falls on a plastic shirt bag in Murdoch's Department Store. She is dressed conservatively—dark blue suit, nice blouse, "sensible" shoes. She falls sideways, landing sharply on her thigh. She lies flat, stunned. A security guard and a clerk, hearing her scream of anguish, rush to see what has happened. The security guard looks down at Sarah. She is not crying out now, but he sees abject terror on her face.

A middle-aged man says, "Don't move her, she could have hurt her spine. Stay still. Don't move anything." Another says, "I'll get help." Sarah does not

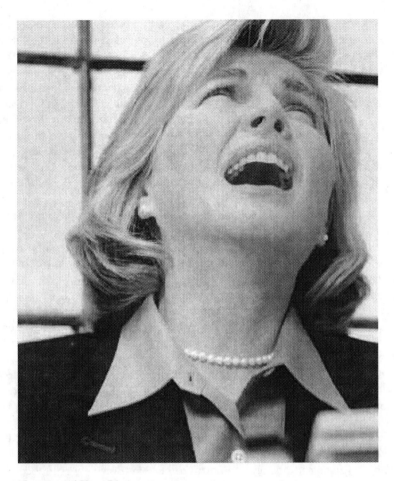

(Courtesy of PhotoDisc)

try to move. She begins to wonder about a numbness in her leg. She cries out, "I can't move my legs. I'm paralyzed. Help me. For God's sake, someone, help me." The clerk assures her that the ambulance has been called. The department manager comes over and asks what has happened. One of the clerks explains, "This woman fell in the aisle. We don't think we should move her until the ambulance arrives." Sarah asks petulantly, "Where is the ambulance? I'm seriously hurt."

Sarah is sure she cannot walk. She feels lightheaded and wonders if she is bleeding internally. The bystanders looking on sense Sarah's concern and reflect it. The manager remembers that any emergency call must be reported to the chief of security.

Arriving quickly on the scene, Alice Turner, the security director, greets Mrs. Paine cordially. Mrs. Paine returns the greeting with a command. "Get me to the hospital. Right now. Call my husband. He's at work. His number is 555-7624. He's the vice president of First National Bank."

In response to the 911 call, Paul Appleton and Sam Peppers arrive within 3 minutes. A security guard points them in Sarah's direction. From the way in which Sarah is lying on the ground, Sam wonders if the fall might have been precipitated by a small stroke or a petit mal seizure. As they near the supine patient, they notice that she is talking steadily to Alice Turner, not allowing Alice much opportunity to respond. She seems to talk very fast, which is perhaps indicative of her anxiety.

Paul recognizes Mrs. Paine. He has treated her before. So have many others at Mercy Ambulance. Once after she was stung by a bee, she drove herself in to the ambulance headquarters, fearing an anaphylactic reaction. The EMS providers introduce themselves. Calmly, Paul asks, "What seems to be wrong?" He almost adds "this time," but he knows this would only cause trouble. He recalls her seemingly endless questions, and he anticipates a similar scene now.

Sarah releases her grip on the store clerk and transfers it to Paul Appleton. She explains that she fell. Her legs seemed to give out underneath her. "It's about time you got here. I must've been lying like this for 15 minutes. I can't move my legs!" Sam explains that as a precaution, he is going to keep her neck still while Paul conducts a thorough assessment. Paul notes the plastic wrapper near her feet. He thinks he has found the cause of her collapse, but to be safe he conducts a thorough assessment. Throughout, Sarah keeps up a round of conversation, despite Sam's admonition to keep still. Paul thinks, "No problem with an open airway here."

Sarah looks at Paul and says, "Young man, you're not listening to me!" Paul is taken aback. The retort was unexpected. It is also true. To Paul's credit, he stops taking vital signs and politely apologizes to her. "I'm sorry, I was preoccupied with my assessment. Right now I need to finish my assessment. Then I'd like to ask a few questions about your medical history while we take care of you."

Alice Turner and another security officer help the EMS providers logroll their patient onto a spine board.

When Paul asks about her medical history, she explains she has been taking aspirin regularly for the past week for muscle pain and headaches. Paul wonders about the possibility of a bleeding disorder complicating the trauma.

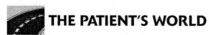 **THE PATIENT'S WORLD**

For a patient such as Mrs. Paine, life revolves around illness and fear of illness. She may be preoccupied with eating right, taking vitamins, avoiding dangerous situations, and keeping regular doctor's appointments. Given an illness situation, hypochondriacal, or somatizing, patients tend to expect the worst. They may know as much or more about health and medical matters as the EMS providers do because they spend a great deal of their time reading medical articles and health books.

THE BEHAVIOR OF THE PATIENT

Two related behaviors are typical with somatizing patients. One is a tendency to focus on symptoms; the second is an attachment to their helpers.

First, a somatizing patient is likely to focus on and exaggerate symptoms and their severity. Mrs. Paine "feels paralyzed." She knows she must go to the emergency department and already fully expects she will be admitted to the hospital. She will act out her symptoms, not consciously obstructing the treatment, but unconsciously confirming her infirmity.

Second, somatizing patients will tend to cling to their helpers, their families, and their friends. Often they will provide complete, detailed medical histories, much of which is not related to the current problem.

THE EMOTIONS AND THOUGHTS BEHIND THE BEHAVIOR

Anxiety and apprehension are the dominant emotions of a somatizing patient. The apprehension Mrs. Paine feels is only loosely linked to her physical injury. She has formulated a worst-case scenario in her mind. If she had a pain in her chest, it would mean an acute myocardial infarction. If she had a cough, it would mean pneumonia or possibly tuberculosis. Her painful ankle becomes a fracture, probably compound, with blood vessel damage. Her inability to move her leg indicates some spinal cord damage. She knew something would happen. The accident has proven her correct.

A great many individuals share Mrs. Paine's concerns. Sometimes this approach to dealing with life is learned in childhood.[2] In some families, parents set up hypochondria by their own behavior. In others, children may learn that illness carries with it secondary gains, such as staying in bed, being cared for, and being relieved of responsibilities. Others may have "learned" from the untimely death of a friend or relative who died from a treatable disease left undiagnosed and untreated. Others may feel they live under a "family death sentence." For example, in a family where men have died of heart attacks in their forties, the expectation of early death is passed on from generation to generation. Finally, for some, disease is a focus in an otherwise unchallenging and empty life.

In adulthood, the person's family may initially support and accommodate to the hypochondriac's behavior. As with victims of chronic disease or depression, there is often a phased response. At first, there is sympathy and understanding.

These feelings then give way to later indifference. Finally, the family may actively avoid the complaining member.

 ## BYSTANDER RESPONSES

A somatizing patient may seek attention and present himself or herself as weaker or more disabled than assessment will show. Among strangers, the somatizing patient may elicit considerable sympathy. Among family, a somatizing patient may evoke many of the same responses that a chronically depressed or suicidal patient can evoke. The family may be burned out by the patient's repeated complaints. Strangers, in contrast, may empathize.

 ## PROVIDER RESPONSES

A somatizing patient, like a chronically depressed patient, can call out indifference in an EMS provider. Just as a family can be burned out, health care providers can be burnt out. Some will tend to ignore reported symptoms as unreliable and exaggerated. Sometimes they feel that by minimizing or downplaying the patient's fears they will help the patient to deal with them. Sometimes, indifference is calculated to show rejection of the patient.

Such a reaction may provide a psychological advantage to a frustrated EMS provider, but it does not serve either the patient or the EMS provider. First, each encounter with a patient must be treated as a new experience. Second, you cannot afford to assume that nothing is wrong with a patient. The old story of the boy who cried wolf provides a tragic example of the results of not listening.

 ## INTERVENTION STRATEGIES

Observe

There will be few observational cues to hypochondria. In fact, looking for these cues can detract from a serious assessment.

Interact

It is very important to take the patient seriously, but not to let the patient's elaborate medical history detract from assessment of the current problem and your care for those problems you have identified. Many times health-care providers make the mistake of assuming that because physical findings are negative, "there's nothing wrong with the patient." Hypochondria and somatization are psychological disorders.

Ask

Unlike a patient who is denying or covering up, the somatizing patient may actually try to run the interview. You may find yourself overwhelmed with facts. If this is the case, you may explain that you have a series of questions you must ask first and that you will welcome further information after you have begun treatment.

Act

Treat the patient as if his or her infirmity is real. It might be!

Attend

As time permits, listen carefully to the patient. A somatizing patient may have a substantial stock of knowledge about the condition and have ideas about proper treatment techniques. Where your protocols may differ from the patient's expectations, you should be able to explain the principles underlying your protocols.

Document

There are no special notes or cautions that apply here, except that derogatory comments about the patient must be avoided. The somatizing patient, like the litigious patient, is more likely than other patients to want copies of medical records.

 ## CONSIDERATIONS FOR EMS PROVIDERS

Attention from a patient like Ms. Harewood can at first be gratifying and then frustrating. A patient like Mr. Hale can make you angry and may make you feel like quitting. A patient like Mrs. Paine can be very frustrating. These difficulties arise from the fact that, in one way or another, these patients violate your expectations. The sexually provocative patient draws you out of your professional role. The litigious patient, consciously or unconsciously, questions your skill and motivation. The somatizing patient seems to mock your ideas about illness by overreacting. Do not take these behaviors personally. Each is rooted in pathology that the emergency situation allows to come to the fore. Recognize that the patient is, in his or her own way, suffering or disadvantaged. Each of these patients may be exasperating; however, it is essential to wait until after you have safely delivered the patient to further care to blow off steam. Even then, a proper respect for the patient requires that you balance your venting with an attempt to seriously imagine what it must be like to walk in the other's shoes.

CONCLUSION

Winston Churchill, who led England during World War II, is reported to have said, "Good judgement comes from experience. Experience comes from bad judgement." Provocative patients who draw attention from the EMS mission to their particular nonmedical needs are an unusual challenge. While such incidents may be rare, understanding patients such as these will help to improve your skill in working with all patients. You are to treat all persons regardless of their background as persons in distress who can benefit from your skilled care.

REVIEW QUESTIONS

1. How might a seductive patient react, verbally or nonverbally, to a focused history and physical examination?
2. How might a litigious patient react, verbally or nonverbally, to a focused history and physical examination?
3. How might a somatizing patient react, verbally or nonverbally, to a focused history and physical examination?
4. How might each of these types of patients attempt to involve bystanders in their situation?

EXERCISES

1. Have an attorney address your group and review the sexual harassment laws.
2. Imagine you are in a place where you do not trust anyone. How might you react?
3. Take a quiet moment and experience all the minor aches and pains in your body (this often increases with age!) Now let your imagination start to find medical causes for each discomfort.
4. Discuss the kinds of unprofessional comments that might appear in documentation.
5. Discuss the ways, if any, a litigious patient should be treated differently from any other patient.

REFERENCES

1. Barry, P. D. (1989). *Psychological nursing assessment and intervention* (2nd ed.) (p. 51). Philadelphia, J. B. Lippincott.

2. Baur, S. (1988). *Hypochondria: woeful imaginings* (p. 54). Berkeley: University of California Press.

FURTHER INFORMATION

Internet Resources

American Law Institute and American Bar Association: www.ali-aba.org/

American Psychiatric Association: www.psych.org

American Psychological Association: www.apa.org

Good law information: www.findlaw.com

Interesting law material (Electric Law Library): www.lectlaw.com

National Association of Mental Health: www.nmha.org

Media Resources

Movies
Erin Brockovich

The Odd Couple

Twelve Angry Men

The Verdict

Books
Foucault, M. (1994). *The birth of the clinic: an archaeology of medical perception.* New York: Random House.

Kerr, B. (1999). *Harmful intent.* New York: Simon & Schuster.

O'Shea, T., & Lalonde, J. (1998). *Sexual harassment: a practical guide to the law, your rights, and your options for taking action.* New York: St. Martin Press.

Slater, L. (2001). *Lying: a metaphorical memoir.* New York: Random House.

Smith, G. R. (1991). *Somatization disorder in the medical setting.* Washington, DC: American Psychiatric Publishing, Inc.

Uribe, C. G. (1999). *The health care providers guide to facing the malpractice deposition.* Boca Raton, FL: CRC Press.

CHAPTER 13

Responding to All People
EMS in the Era of Diversity

OBJECTIVES

Upon completion of this chapter, you should be able to:

- Identify ways in which the United States has become an increasingly diverse nation.
- List the various types of diversity.
- Demonstrate the power and dangers of stereotypes and prejudice.
- Differentiate between prejudice and discrimination.
- Show ways to deal with your own and the community's prejudices.

THE CHALLENGE

America is a richly diverse nation, and that diversity includes sex, religion, race, ethnic origin, geographic region, sexual orientation, and persons with disabilities—both physical and mental. People from all over the world come to stay in the United States. Box 13–1 summarizes the percentages of various ethnic groups living in the United States. They come from Africa, Europe, the Middle East, Asia, India, South America, Central America, and Australia. They bring with them their religions. So, in addition to Catholic, Protestant, and Jewish faiths, our religious tapestry now includes other major world religions such as Islam, Hinduism, and Buddhism. Americans have many different orientations.

EMS providers are challenged to come to grips with their own prejudices and to deal with the prejudices of the very people to whom they are responding. The best way to proceed is to define the terms *stereotyping, prejudice, ethnocentricity,* and *discrimination.*

BOX 13–1

PROJECTED PERCENTAGE OF THE U.S. POPULATION IN 2006

White	69.5%
Hispanic	12.8%
African American	12.4%
Asian	4.5%
Native American	0.8%

Source: Thio, A. (1998). *Sociology* (5th ed.). New York: Harper Collins.

Stereotyping means seeing all people of a certain group—whether they be Latin American or Jewish or Asian—in a certain way. Stereotyping looks at members of ethnic and religious groups as all behaving the same way and does *not* recognize individual differences and variations. **Prejudice** involves seeing others who are different from you as inferior.[1] **Ethnocentricity** involves seeing one's own group's culture and values as superior to all others. Therefore, an ethnocentric person views the culture and values of other groups as inferior.[2]

Discrimination involves action not just attitude. A discriminator acts on the basis of ethnocentric and prejudiced attitudes. Discrimination is often supported by custom and law. It means acting on your prejudices. For example, John Doe may believe that all gays are promiscuous. This is his opinion. However, when John refuses to rent to or hire a gay person because of that individual's sexual orientation, that is discrimination.

The ultimate challenge is *not* prejudice, stereotyping, and ethnocentrism. These exist. The real test is in recognizing and working with these attitudes as professionals (Box 13–2). Although textbooks frequently admonish students and practitioners to be nonjudgmental in their approach to patients, this is easier said than done. It is far more useful to acknowledge the feelings and then *not* to allow them to interfere with our response and responsibilities.

BOX 13–2

SIGNIFICANCE FOR EMS

EMS personnel are themselves a diverse professional group responding to medical emergencies occurring in an increasingly diverse population.

THE PATIENT AND THE SITUATION

Allison Wentworth adjusts the mirror, puts on the lights and siren, and tells her partner Rodney Jefferson Roosevelt to get the water wings ready "because we're off to Puerto Rico." He leans back as Allison announces the mission to respond to Anita Rodriguez's labor pains. This run means once again entering the area called Little Puerto Rico and seeing if Anita is really in labor. Neither of them like or look forward to the run. The neighborhood has been less than welcoming and each has mental baggage from prior runs. Each silently prepares for another "English as a second language encounter" and wonders if there will be a father there.

Allison grew up in northern New England. She comes from a stoic tradition and has always been slightly annoyed by the screaming of Hispanic women in labor. Although she has taken many courses in psychology and sociology, she still does not understand why people can't control their emotions. She also believes, as an individual concerned about the environment, that there should only be two children per family and is therefore bothered by any large family.

Meanwhile, Rodney, an African American, remembers all too vividly the "warfare" in Chicago between Latino gangs and Black gangs. Hence, he anticipates an encounter with an overprotective and defensive male. He feels a slight adrenaline rush as they accelerate. He wonders if this run will be to help a pregnant woman or to defend himself.

On the sidewalk leading to the apartment, the EMS providers are greeted by a man in a suit and tie waving to them from 13 Columbia Way. Allison parks the vehicle and they proceed toward the apartment. As they approach the unit, they detect a singularly unhappy expression on the man's face. He identifies himself as Juan Rodriguez and asks provocatively, "What took you so long?" Before

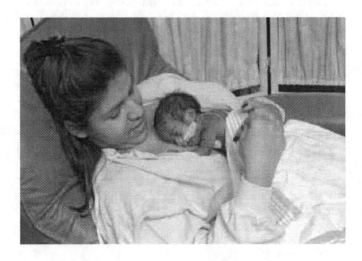

either EMS provider can answer he shouts, "How come the city does not send Latinos to this neighborhood?" and "Why aren't you taking care of my wife?" Suddenly, Allison and Rodney realize that all of their prejudices and stereotypes pale next to this man's.

However, before Juan and the two EMS providers have a chance to square off against one another, all hear a warm, quiet, slightly panicked woman's voice from inside the apartment—"Here comes the pain again—will someone please help me!" A look of concern on Juan Rodriguez's face rouses them from their world of preconceptions and they start to address the reason they are all there—to help Anita Rodriguez deliver a healthy baby. They work together to transport her to Cedars of Lebanon Hospital. There she delivers a beautiful 8 pound 5 ounce baby boy with an Apgar score of 10. Juan shakes Rodney's hand, gives him a cigar, and hugs Allison. Allison with a hint of tears in her eyes walks away, feeling good about helping to bring a new life into this world.

 ## THE PATIENT'S WORLD

If you are a member of a majority group you must be ready to let go of your preconceptions to understand the position of a minority patient in this situation. You must put yourself in the place of a person whose culture and experiences with the health-care system may be very different from your own. For many members of minority populations, the patient's world is dominated by feelings of alienation, fear, apprehension, and danger.

Indeed, many folks have come to America seeking a refuge as the Statue of Liberty proclaims—"Give me your tired, huddled masses yearning to be free." They may have come from war-torn environments where uniforms meant arrest, torture, and death. For many refugees, the sound of certain sirens can bring back memories of arrest and dislocation. So for them you may not represent help and hope but rather yet another symbol of dreaded power and enforcement. Granted this is an extreme situation, but it allows you to start to see the world in a new and different light.

Consider some examples of what minority members may experience daily. Public safety officers detain an African-American accountant as he drives home late at night in his BMW through a very nice suburban town. A woman is furious with both her employer who pays her less than men doing the same job and her devoted husband who still loves to call her the "little woman." A Latino couple are refused a room at a motel that becomes suddenly full as they approach the desk. An obese woman finds coworkers laughing at her behind her back. A Philippine emigrant is only given janitorial work despite his college education. An Asian student is told "I think it's amazing the way you people are so good in math," by a landlord when he looks at an apartment. A white man complains that he cannot get a job because the company only wants to hire minorities to enhance its diversified image. Stereotypes, prejudice, and past discrimination set up expectations that influence future behavior.

 ## THE BEHAVIOR OF THE PATIENT

A patient's responses to a lifetime of perceived humiliation and second-class citizenship are many and varied. Many will cooperate with authority. Some take on a belligerent stance and jump in ready for a confrontation as Juan Rodriguez did. They fight fire with fire. Still others will simply avoid contact with those in power. They will live, love, and work within their own community. Another group will actually become self-loathing and incorporate what they believe to be the majority view of themselves. For example, a rather large man showered twice a day so he would smell right.

 ## THE EMOTIONS AND THOUGHTS BEHIND THE BEHAVIOR

Patient behavior reflects a wide range of conflicting emotions and ideas about being a member of a minority group. For many there is the sense of shame of not being included and humiliation of not being considered good enough. They may acknowledge that they will never be in the seat of power and be in control. These beliefs lead to smoldering feelings of depression, alienation, and helplessness. Others take the same sense of being on the outside and draw energy from it. This feeling of alienation can then go in one of two ways. Some will work with the system to gain power over time. Others will go outside the system and use criminal means to succeed.

Another group will adopt a helpless attitude. They have never been listened to, feel victimized by the majority, and have a sense of being oppressed. This behavior has been called **learned helplessness**.[3] These persons have found that however they respond, they either have been punished or have failed. They have learned to feel and act helpless.

Others will find a sense of group pride as a counterattitude to the majority. Gay pride and Black power provide dramatic examples of this. This feeling of pride can be fueled by hatred and manipulated by leaders. Yet, more often, being proud of one's identity allows expression of positive values—love of family and community and cherishing one's heritage and traditions.

If you appreciate ethnic, religious, cultural geographic, racial, sexual identity, and sources of group pride, you can now understand one of the greatest paradigm shifts in Americans' view of themselves. Historically, America was noted to be a **melting pot**. Hence, people from all over the world would come here and in the great caldron of this country fuse together. This fusion did not work because certain groups never fused and many groups did not want to lose their identify. A new concept of diversity has emerged—the **tossed salad** idea. America is made up of many groups—tomatoes, cucumbers, lettuce, and radishes. Each flavor contributes to the whole, yet each remains distinct.

 FAMILY/BYSTANDER RESPONSES

The responses of the family and bystanders will significantly affect the EMS intervention. Family members are in a pivotal position to influence both the patient and the professional treatment. Indeed, they can act in one of three distinct roles: *preventing help, passively blocking care,* or *encouraging assistance.* Let us look at each of these situations.

Preventing Help

Returning to the Rodriguez's family story, imagine if the neighbors all shared Juan's rage, hostility, and confrontational attitude toward the EMS providers. Had the family and bystanders been caught up in their anger, they could have delayed or even prevented care and transport. In extreme situations, EMS providers have had to wait for police backup before entering certain neighborhoods.

Passively Blocking Care

In a less radical but perhaps equally vexing way, the family and bystanders remain uninvolved because of their indifference to the situation. In one situation, EMS providers were responding to a woman in labor who was hemorrhaging. They initially attended her in her second-story bedroom. The huge extended family continued to watch a television show as the staff brought her out on a gurney. Their TV viewing obstructed the intervention.

Encouraging Assistance

Consider what would happen if Juan had a less angry neighbor, relative, or friend who might have suggested to him that the needs of his wife outweighed his wrath. Very often a good friend or family member can gently take the person aside and allow EMS treatment. There are Samaritans in many cases and they do make a difference. Anita Rodriguez became that voice of reason in a turmoil sea of stereotypes and prejudice.

 PROVIDER RESPONSES

EMS providers in responding to a patient who is different than themselves must keep in mind several key principles: *recognize your own feelings but act professionally; remember the diversity paradox;* and *treat the patient as you would expect your mother to be treated.* The reason for these ideas remains that you work in an ever-expanding, diversified world. America is no longer the neat Normal Rockwell *Saturday Evening Post* pictures. You are working in a salad not a melting pot!

Recognize your own feelings but act professionally. Each responding EMS provider has his and her own feelings and reactions to others. Many are very tolerant. Others have moments when they fulfill a stereotype. Certainly, Allison has a stoic heritage. She handles life and its stresses differently than others would. That is the way she deals with crisis. Similarly, Rodney has his own issues. The fights of his youth rage in his head. That is his background expectation. We do not expect them to be saints nor even to be totally nonjudgmental. But we can and do expect them to be professional at all times during the intervention. During World War II, a Jewish physician operated successfully on a Nazi officer. When asked how he could perform such surgery he replied that the patient was a *"wounded man and I am a doctor."*

Remember the diversity paradox. It is a strange double truth of diversity literature: everyone is both similar to others and everyone is different. Everyone regardless of race, religion, ethic origin, sexual preference, and mental and physical challenges does need security, satisfaction of physical needs, respect, love, and the opportunity to show his or her care for children and others. Yes, we are all part of the human family! We vary in our mental and physical capacities and pursue these wishes in a vast array of different ways. However, our expectations are shaped by our experiences as members of specific groups: racial, religious, ethnic, and sexual preference. And, of course, even within these groups were are a wide variety of expressions. Just look at the wide variety of ways Christians worship Christ. Look at the varying dietary laws of the different faiths. Yes, we all eat, but we eat in such different ways!

Treat the patient as you would expect your mother to be treated. If you have any doubt as to the care you are providing, remember this rule. How *would* you expect and hope EMS providers would care for your loved ones. Yes, people are diverse and some are very different, but just ask yourself how you would want your family to be treated.

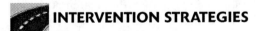 **INTERVENTION STRATEGIES**

Observe

The best way to observe the patient and the scene is with an open mind. Again, this is easier said than done. When Allison and Rodney encountered Juan, they stereotyped him as a "typical macho Latino male." Certainly, he did present himself as arrogant and confrontational. Yet, because of their assumptions, they may have missed the worried, concerned husband and father-to-be underneath the verbal volcano (Box 13–3).

As you work with patients and their families it is always useful to remember that *assume makes an ass of you and me.* How many times have you made a hasty decision and jumped to an erroneous conclusion? Many of us in our quick judgment put our feet in our months.

Interact

Communication across racial and ethnic groups is complicated by the various assumptions different cultures make about appropriate behavior. These assumptions include active listening behavior; use of translators; understanding the three ways people communicate face to face; and an appreciation for interpersonal space.

Active listening means listening to what the patient and the family are saying. Again, easier said than done. When people do not speak English or when they have trouble communicating because of a physical or emotional challenge, it can be very difficult to understand the meaning behind the words. Give the patient or family the time to get their ideas out. Show them you are trying to understand them. Ask family and friends to help you comprehend what they are saying. One patient with cerebral palsy had great difficulty in articulating what was wrong and where the pain was. Yet, a persistent, caring EMS provider was slowly able to decipher the patient's message and concerns.

Use a translator if necessary. What does dealing with a deaf person, helping an individual who only speaks Russian, working with a Japanese patient who does not speak English, and assisting a Navaho man who can only talk in his ancient tongue have in common? In each case the patient has great difficulty in communicating with EMS providers. Each situation requires a translator. Again, easier said than done. If the encounter occurs in a hospital during working hours and not under emergency conditions, then the written and postprocedure involves obtaining a listed translator.

Incorporating that procedure in the field is a challenge but can be done. Ask family and friends for help. Draw on the neighborhood expertise and experiences. Call for a backup translator.

Be aware that face-to-face communication is done three ways. When two people talk face to face, they communicate in three ways simultaneously: verbally, through tone of voice, and through body language. This transmission of information happens regardless of ethnic or racial or any other cultural differences. Furthermore, body language and tone are more important than words in conveying information. Experts estimate that we receive 70 percent of our information in face-to-face communication through body language; 23 percent through tone of voice; and only 7 percent through the words that are used.[4] Therefore, be aware at all times that you are communicating in three ways. For example, Juan may hear Allison's words, "We are here to help," but her tone of voice is one of disgust and her body language suggests disdain. So Juan sees and hears different messages.

Cultural differences increase the opportunity for distortion and misunderstanding. For example, in the United States looking someone straight in the eye suggests interest and honesty. Yet, for many Asians, avoiding eye contact shows respect.

Appreciate interpersonal space. In many interventions, EMS providers will benefit by paying attention to the patient's or bystander's comfort zones. In some cultures people routinely speak to each other at closer distances than do most North Americans. This closeness can feel very uncomfortable. In other cultures, people expect more personal space. Remember that our ideas about appropriate personal space are culturally conditioned. There is no right or wrong distance. When someone "gets in our face," we may feel uncomfortable and angry. However, different cultures have different ideas about what distance is too close. Being too close to an angry patient may further provoke him and antagonize the crisis. For example, standing too close to Juan would be a huge error in communication. Respecting interpersonal space is indicated in certain circumstances. When delivering lifesaving care, as in bleeding control and resuscitation situations, EMS providers can still demonstrate their respect for the patient in the explanations they provide and the professionalism with which they move.

Ask

Asking patients and families relevant medical questions represents a very important part of the assessment in all emergencies. In all cases EMS providers must be sensitive in how they are making the inquiries. However, EMS providers must be particularly vigilant and sensitive when asking questions of individuals from different cultural backgrounds. There are a number of useful inquiry techniques that will both enhance the quality of the information obtained and make the patient and family comfortable. Begin with a sense of respect for the person you are securing information from and incorporate the concepts developed in the "Interact" section.

It remains critical in the inquiry process to convey the sense of respect for the patient and the family and treat them with dignity. For example, an EMS crew had to transport Mr. Won Lee, an 82-year-old Chinese man, to the hospital. When they called him "Won," they did not show respect. When they brushed past family members and whisked him onto the stretcher, their body language did not indicate caring or concern. Patients and families from many different groups distrust authorities. Hence, they will be paying particular attention not only to the words of the questions but also to your tone of voice and body language.

Again, for all patients but especially in these situations, explaining the reason for the question helps to secure cooperation and involvement. Reminding the persons being served of the medical rationale for the inquiry makes them more comfortable. Reiterating that you ask all people in these situations the same questions may ease their concerns. And, of course, observing proper interpersonal distances avoids your being in their face and being threatening to them.

Act

Here, as in all situations, EMS providers should tell people in advance the actions they plan to take and the reasons for those actions. For example, a 10-year-old Cambodian girl had an acute abdomen—probably appendicitis. The EMS providers were concerned to get to the hospital as swiftly as possible. In their haste, they did not inform the parents and the neighbors of their plan. The gathered community became very agitated when they thought the child was being kidnapped.

Attend

In addition to attending the patient as in all emergencies, it is important to remember to include the family in the transport. Family members can help reassure the patient and also serve as translators.

Document

Document as in all cases but remember to avoid any terms or descriptions that could be interpreted as prejudicial or as stereotyping the patient and the community. Box 13–4 summarizes "Intervention Strategies" when working with patients of various cultures.

BOX 13–4

STRATEGY

Observe	be aware of others' differences and similarities
Interact	listen to what they are saying; use translators to facilitate communication; be aware of the three ways to communicate
Ask	respectfully with concern in order to understand
Act	not only medically but with sensitivity to others' traditions
Attend	stay with the patient
Document	record times, interventions, medications without comment

CONSIDERATIONS FOR EMS PROVIDERS

What does diversity mean to EMS providers? The answer is, a great deal. The heart of the consideration remains that America is an evermore diverse nation. We see increasing diversity in our towns and cities, in our schools and workplaces, and in our places of worship. Directly for EMS providers diversity represents two critical realities—the person you are riding with is more likely to be *different* from you and the individual you are treating is more likely to be *different* from you.

Therefore, each EMS provider must not only appreciate the new world he or she is working in but also must understand his or her own prejudices. In the final analysis you must deliver a professional intervention. Being respectful, sensitive, and self-insightful leads to a better intervention.

CONCLUSION

Most people who were born and raised in the United States have a shared understanding of the role of police officers, firefighters, and EMS providers. People who grew up in other cultures and members of some American subcultures do not necessarily share these understandings. In many parts of the world, people do not expect police to be well trained or fair; these views may sometimes transfer to their dealings with EMS.

REVIEW QUESTIONS

1. How has the population of the United States of America changed in the last 10 years?
2. Define stereotype, prejudice, and discrimination.
3. How do EMS provider's prejudices affect their work?
4. List several techniques EMS providers can use both to improve communication and to comfort patients from different backgrounds.

EXERCISES

1. List the various cultures and groups you belong to.
2. Invite members or representatives from various communities; for example, African American, Latino, Asian, or Gay and Lesbian, to discuss their cultures and their experiences with the EMS System.
3. Visit an ethnic neighborhood. Walk around, eat in its restaurants, and attend a worship service there.

4. Watch a movie depicting racism and then discuss it.

5. Discuss how the population in your community has changed in the last 10 years.

6. Discuss what you think leads people in a community to distrust EMS providers.

REFERENCES

1. Carr-Ruffino, N. (1996). *Managing diversity: people skills for a multicultural workplace.* Thomson Executive Press.

2. Thio, A. (1998). *Sociology.* (5th ed.). New York: Harper Collins.

3. Kaplan, H. I., Sadock, B. J., & Grebb, J. A. (1994). *Kaplan and Sadock's synopsis of psychiatry* (7th ed.). Baltimore: Williams & Wilkins.

4. Tamparo, C. D., & Wilburta, Q. L. (2002). *Therapeutic communications for allied health professionals* (2nd ed.). Clifton Park, NY: Delmar Learning.

FURTHER INFORMATION

Internet Resources

www.inform.umd.edu/EdRes/Topic/Diversity

Guess Who's Coming to Dinner, Teach with Movies Learning Guide provides a series of questions that can be used to spark discussion about some of the racial themes brought up in this 1967 film: www.teachwithmovies.org

Diversity Training Products: www.hrpress-diversity.com

Media Resources

Movies
American History X

Apt Pupil

Dances with Wolves

Driving Miss Daisy

Once Were Warriors

A Raisin in the Sun

Remember the Titans

Roots (television series)

A Soldier's Story

Thelma and Louise

Books

Adams, M., Blumenfeld, W. J., Castenada, R., Hackman, H. W., Peters, M. L., & Zuniga, X. (Eds.). (2000). *Readings for diversity and social justice: an anthology on racism, sexism, classism, anti-semitism, heterosexism, and ableism.* New York: Routledge.

Bucher, R. D. (1999). *Diversity consciousness: opening our minds to people, cultures, and opportunities.* Upper Saddle River, NJ: Prentice Hall.

Carroll, S. B., Weatherbee, S. D., & Grenier, J. K. (2000). *From DNA to diversity.* Oxford, UK: Blackwell Science.

Luckman, J. (2000). *Transcultural communication in health care.* Clifton Park, NY: Delmar Learning.

Thomas, T. R. (1999). *Building a house for diversity: how a fable about a giraffe and elephant offers new strategies for today's workforce.* New York: AMACOM.

CHAPTER 14

Death in the Ambulance
Grief and Guilt

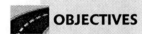 **OBJECTIVES**

Upon completion of this chapter, you should be able to:

- Reflect on your own attitude toward death.
- Understand some of the concerns of family and friends regarding death.
- Explain the grieving process and how it might relate to the behavior of the patient's family.
- Demonstrate how you might respond to a family after a patient has died while in your care.

THE CHALLENGE

Emergency care has changed. People's expectations of ambulance service have changed. Instead of considering it an expensive taxi, most people recognize the ambulance as an extension of the medical center.

A death in the ambulance can be a devastating experience. Initially, it may result in an awkward conversation with a survivor. Later it may lead to second guessing and guilt. If an EMS provider's feelings about death are not resolved, they can lead to burnout. Death is a part of life. Most deaths that occur in the field will be beyond the ability of the EMS provider to prevent. In some cases, there will be real questions as to whether all that could have been done was done. Whatever the case, dealing with death is one of the most profound challenges an EMS provider will face. Further, it is one that most experienced EMS providers will face.

To meet the challenge of death in the ambulance, the EMS providers must be there for the patient and the patient's family. To fully meet the challenge, however, they must be there for each other as well.

THE PATIENT AND THE SITUATION

At 6:30 A.M., 57-year-old Bernard Gorham wakes from an uneasy sleep. He is gasping for breath. He feels as if a steel hoop is tightening around his chest, preventing the expansion of his lungs. He cannot get air in. Helen, his wife of 32 years, does not panic. She recognizes his bouts of respiratory distress as painful but manageable. In fact, Bernard is scheduled for a radiological exam at the Whitman Medical Center this morning. The ambulance has been called for 8:00 A.M.

Bernard leans forward and braces himself, placing his arms against the top of the night table. Helen turns on the oxygen beside the bed, adjusts the flow meter to 4 liters per minute, and places the prongs of the cannula gently into his nostrils.

She pats Bernard gently on the arm, as she has done countless times before, and calls Mercy Ambulance to ask if they could arrive a little bit earlier because her husband seems very uncomfortable. She wants him checked out in the emergency department (ED) before the x-ray, but she doesn't see any reason to bother Dr. Janet Kellog at this hour of the morning. In fact, Mercy Ambulance and the ED personnel know Bernard well. Just in case Bernard is admitted for observation, she packs his overnight bag with a fresh pair of pajamas, toothbrush, razor, comb, and the mystery novel he has been reading.

She wakes their two teenage children who live at home. Jessica, age 16, is a high school student, and William, age 18, is a student at the local community college. This morning they will stay behind to take their mother to the hospital. They accept their father's chronic illness as a part of their lives. Bernard's lungs have been compromised due to his occupational exposure to silica dust while working as a sandblaster. The fact that he was a two-pack-a-day smoker contributed to his impairment.[1]

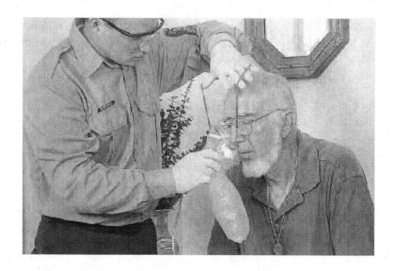

Now on disability, he has had to restrict activity markedly in the past several months. It used to be that he could help around the house and babysit his oldest son's toddler. Now the little boy is too active for him, and even routine household chores must be restricted. The grandfather clock at the bottom of the stairs strikes 7 o'clock as Jessica wolfs down a quick breakfast. She has a fleeting memory of the old song "My Grandfather's Clock" as it chimes.

The Mercy Ambulance dispatcher knows the Gorhams well. He tries to accommodate their desires. Mrs. Gorham is a pleasant woman, and her husband, for all his pain, is very cooperative with the EMS providers. The dispatcher is always impressed with how matter-of-factly she deals with her husband's difficulties. Betty Eastford and John Paulson have just signed in at Mercy Ambulance. They had expected to pick up Mr. Gorham at 8:00 A.M., but will, at his wife's request, arrive earlier.

At 7:25 the ambulance arrives at the Gorhams' house. Bernard has adapted his life-style to his illness. Betty and John are grateful that he has moved the master bedroom to the first floor of the cape-style house. He breathes with great difficulty. When he sees the ambulance crew, recognition and appreciation show in his eyes. For just a second, but an important second, the anticipated help eases his discomfort. He is thankful that it is Betty and John and not that new kid who was so rough. Betty and John greet him and begin their assessment. His pulse is 122 and irregular. His respirations are 32 and shallow, with oxygen running. His blood pressure is 110/90. Bernard cooperates in the examination but does not attempt to speak.

Carefully, they lift Bernard on the stretcher, secure him, and set up their oxygen before moving him to the ambulance. They confirm that they will meet Mrs. Gorham and her children at the Whitman Hospital ED. Betty attends to Bernard in the back, while John drives in the early rush hour traffic.

Bernard's difficulty intensifies. Betty notes that he relies more on accessory muscles for breathing, and she feels his radial pulse become weaker. She increases the oxygen flow.

Her eyes meet his. The glimmer of recognition is gone. Instead, she finds a strange, vacant look. She feels a thready, very rapid carotid pulse. "John," she calls, "I've lost a pulse." "I'm starting CPR!" She lowers the stretcher, loosens the straps, and quickly places a spine board behind Bernard's back. Her eyes meet his. This time, however, she is startled to realize he is not looking back at her. John accelerates, turns on lights and siren, and cuts through the traffic. Betty has a strange feeling. John radios ahead to Whitman that they have an arrest en route. Theoretically, Bernard Gorham is still alive. Betty continues CPR. She has no way of knowing what the monitor will show, but she feels deeply that it will be a flat line, not ventricular fibrillation.

At the Whitman ED, Dr. Wilkinson, a busy young intern, begins a code, but calls it short after the electrocardiogram (ECG) confirms Betty's instinct. He is tired, and appears somewhat cynical. Dr. Wilkinson pronounces death at 7:50

A.M. However, he asks Betty and John if they know Bernard's religion. John assumes he is a Catholic because of the Madonna in a small grotto in the front yard. The charge nurse in the ED calls the Catholic chaplain.

John and Betty support each other. Yet, she has nagging doubts. Neither questions what they did once Mr. Gorham's condition turned for the worse. Rather, they worry that they missed an important assessment clue or failed to notice his deterioration early enough. They wonder if they spent too much time at the house. Betty wonders if she should have paid more attention to Mr. Gorham on the ride to the hospital.

Betty stares vacantly at the run record. It is trivial, but she realizes how little information they collected. The blankness of the insurance section stands out starkly. She can't talk about that with Mrs. Gorham now. "The family! Oh God, I forgot about the family," she thinks. They will be arriving any minute expecting to find Bernard going to radiology.

At 7:54 A.M., Helen, Jessica, and William Gorham arrive. Betty points them out to the charge nurse, who quickly ushers them into a quiet room. William guesses that this is typical treatment to separate families from sick people. Helen feels uneasy: she has never been treated this way before. She shivers visibly at the thought that something is wrong—very wrong.

The charge nurse literally pushes Dr. Wilkinson into the room, with scant warning that the family is here. The intern knew Bernard Gorham only as an unshaven corpse on an ambulance cot. He pauses awkwardly, ". . . Mrs. . . . Gorham, I'm Dr. Wilkinson. I'm sorry. Your husband's heart failed in the ambulance. They did all that they could for him, but . . . I'm very sorry."

Hearing that short, hurried apology, the family disintegrates. William wants to hit someone—the doctor, the charge nurse, the ambulance crew. Someone is responsible for this! Dr. Wilkinson, adds, "The chaplain would like to see you," as he heads for the door. Helen taps an inner strength she has always known was there. She fully expected that Bernie's time was limited and knew that he would not last forever. But this morning? This time? She really was unprepared. Her concern for William and for Jessica keeps her steady. She thanks the "fleeing" doctor, shielding him from her son's rage.

Betty and John have been in the doorway during this brief drama. Both are moved. Betty comes forward to express her sympathy to Mrs. Gorham. "Mr. Gorham was very brave. He was always kind and considerate to us." Mrs. Gorham thanks her. John is more reticent. He is clearly uncomfortable with the subject of death. He mutters, "I'm very sorry about your husband." He realizes that nothing he says will be sufficient but that he must say something. The charge nurse comes in to announce that Dr. Kellog is on the telephone and that the chaplain would like to have a word with Mrs. Gorham and her children.

Betty and John leave quietly. If the billing office wants to collect on this run, let them get the insurance information.

THE PATIENT'S WORLD

Every death, like every life, is individual. Nevertheless, there are two general considerations that will shape the experience. First, there is the history of the patient. Second, there are religious and cultural factors.

The history of the patient—especially experience with chronic or near-fatal disease or injury in the past—can affect his or her current view. Some patients, even though the present illness has developed rapidly, may be prepared for death by previous experiences. For example, one man suffering chest pain that radiated down his left arm knew he was having a heart attack. Instead of being overwhelmed by the experience, he reported being ready for it: he had accepted death after he had suffered his first heart attack 20 years before and had lived his life to the fullest since then.

Religious and cultural factors are especially important in shaping the response to death. A belief in heaven, or in reincarnation, shapes the experience of death for believers. Death has replaced sex as a taboo subject for many people, however, and may arouse tremendous anxiety.

 ## THE BEHAVIOR OF THE PATIENT

Kübler-Ross has identified five stages that patients go through when dying: denial, anger, bargaining, depression, and acceptance (see Box 14–1).[2] Denial means they do not acknowledge they have a fatal illness. They often seek second and third opinions. Anger represents their frustration and rage that they are dying. They want to do things, have places to go; they do not want to die. Bargaining involves the process in which patients offer things they would do or

---

BOX 14–1

KÜBLER-ROSS' FIVE STAGES OF DYING

1. *Denial*   Refuses to acknowledge there is a problem

2. *Anger*   Is angered easily; may take it out on caregivers

3. *Bargaining*   Makes deals in hopes of prolonging life

4. *Depression*   Withdraws from family; wants to be left alone

5. *Acceptance*   Puts things in order, says goodbye

Source: *On death and dying*, by E. Kübler-Ross, 1970, New York: Macmillan. Copyright 1970 by Macmillan.

be if death could be delayed or avoided. For example, some say they would go to church more or be better parents. Then there is depression. Here, patients appreciate the losses—no more watching the children or grandchildren grow, no more being with family and friends, and just no more being. In this stage, the full feelings of sadness occur. Finally, many people reach a level of acceptance. They accept and even greet and welcome their deaths. Some patients will not go through the entire process; others may progress and then return to another phase. Some will go through the five stages.

THE EMOTIONS AND THOUGHTS BEHIND THE BEHAVIOR

In considering emotions and thoughts, it is important to consider the patient's state at a particular time, as well as the stage of dying at which you encounter him. The person's mood at the time of the illness or crisis can be a factor. A person who is "down"—not chronically depressed, but at a low point, psychologically—may see life as wasted or meaningless at that moment and accept death. This may not be his characteristic view, but it will be real to him at that moment. At the other extreme, a patient who is "up" may be angry, or bargaining, feeling that he or she is being cheated of new opportunities.

FAMILY/BYSTANDER RESPONSES

When the death in the ambulance is unexpected, the survivors are forced to confront their loss without adequate preparation. The grief over the loss can be overwhelming, and the behavior of the survivors can seem totally inexplicable. Responses can include grief, anger, depression, self-deprecation, and physical pain.

The Gorhams were not prepared to hear that their husband and father had died. It was unexpected. They had had no time to say goodbye. Even worse, he died alone. Yes, he was attended, but he died among strangers, and he died within reach of the hospital.

A family can react to such a death in a number of ways. Most will utter an audible gasp. In the ED, this sound inevitably indicates that a survivor has heard of a death for the first time. It is a sound of anguish and despair, which will stay with those who hear it for the rest of their lives.

Generally, behavior may represent some way of fleeing the messenger or fighting the messenger. Some survivors become rigid, paralyzed, or catatonic in response to the news. Others drop to the floor. Others threaten the physician or nurse who brought the news, sometimes with physical force. Some will walk away alone; others will cling to friends and relatives. The reaction may include physical symptoms. Sometimes these symptoms will mimic the symptoms reported by the deceased. For example, one survivor, on hearing that his older brother had died of a heart attack, experienced severe pain in his own chest.

Some will experience frustration, anger, and rage. This may be directed toward God, the hospital, the last people to treat the loved one, or others who are somehow seen as responsible.

A series of thoughts will sweep through the survivor's mind. In no particular order, the survivor may remember what the deceased did earlier that day, their last meal together, their last embrace, some small kindness, and so forth. This mental flooding can generate doubt and guilt. "Should I have called the doctor? Did I wait too long? Did I miss something that I should have seen?" Similar doubts may come to haunt the EMS providers as well.

Over the next few days, social customs dictate a grieving process that may include a wake and funeral. Specific responses will depend on the deceased's past history and relationship with the family, and the family's cultural and religious context.

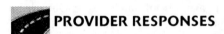 ## PROVIDER RESPONSES

The EMS providers' experience of a patient dying on their watch has many similarities to the experience of the family. Betty Eastford and John Paulson, riding on to the rest of the day's responsibilities, sense the loss of a man. They had participated in the moment of death and then in that painful moment when the family heard the news. They also have nagging doubts about their performance. Did their care contribute to Mr. Gorham's death? Did Betty and John adequately assess his condition, or did they assume, because it was a scheduled run, that Mr. Gorham was OK? They took all the proper measures, but did they really interpret them? Should they have recognized that he needed more care than they could provide? Should they have called for advanced life support? Later at the hospital, should they have said more to Mrs. Gorham, Jessica, and William?

An EMS provider can develop a strong appreciation and understanding of a patient in a relatively short time. In contrast to the impression many texts would give, the relationship between EMS provider and patient is *not* one between two strangers. At times of crisis, people may not say much, but what they say is very revealing.

In some cases, especially with volunteers in smaller communities, the EMS providers may know the patient as a personal friend. We know of one case in which a teacher who volunteered with the local squad found herself transporting one of her pupils to the hospital after a fatal accident that had already claimed the life of the child's parents. She was nearly overwhelmed with emotion but still did the job, getting the child to the hospital. Yet, this is the type of incident that must be worked through; preferably through an established critical incident stress debriefing (CISD) program. Where CISD resources are not available, a trained psychotherapist or pastoral counselor may be helpful.

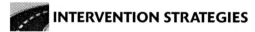 **INTERVENTION STRATEGIES**

Observe

Your initial observations—even before you know or suspect that your patient may be dying—will provide valuable clues to appropriate behavior with the individual and his family. In general, your observations should include any important features of the patient's environment that might be important for treatment. In addition, look for obvious indications of religious affiliation and family connections. If there are pets that might go uncared for, a note to hospital social services or an animal welfare agency is appropriate.

Where it is obvious that the patient is not resuscitatable, you should know and follow local ambulance service protocols. It is critical that you are familiar with state and local laws and regulations concerning CPR and Do Not Resuscitate statutes. They vary from area to area and from state to state. Document carefully your reasons for not initiating treatment. You should be familiar with the reasons for not initiating CPR recognized by the American Heart Association. In the case of a possible homicide or suicide victim, again follow ambulance service policies, which should be consistent with those of the local police.

Interact

It is easy to forget that comatose patients or stroke patients can often hear even though they cannot speak or respond. An EMS provider, trapped in his car after a collision with another vehicle, vividly recalled snatches of conversation as he drifted in and out of consciousness. Worst of all, he could sense the activity around him but could not make sense of it.[3] His greatest relief came from hearing his rescuers explain what they were doing. This was the only way he knew he had not been given up for dead. If the patient dies, show proper respect for the body. It is a time for reverence, not morbid humor.

Interaction with family members, if they are present, is especially important. There are four key points to effective communication. These are summarized in Box 14–2. First, whenever possible, keep the family informed of the patient's medical status during the intervention. In certain states, the EMS providers do not pronounce a patient dead, but in all cases they can provide care information to the family. Many ED trauma teams designate a member to tell the family what is happening. In our scenario, there was no way that Betty could have kept the family informed. The sudden announcement of death at the hospital was unexpected. Second, code words, buzz words, and shop talk can be troubling to a family at any time but never more than when spoken at the side of a dying patient. Third, families usually value hearing that all that

---

BOX 14-2

EMT RESPONSIBILITIES TO THE FAMILY

- Keep family members informed of the patient's status.
- Avoid buzz words and shop talk.
- Assure the family that all that could have been done was done and, if appropriate, let the family know that the patient did not suffer.
- Recognize that family members will respond out of their own emotions and thoughts, which may have little to do with what you have done.

---

could be done was done and that the patient did not suffer. Assuming that these statements are true, they bear reinforcing to the family.

Fourth, you must recognize that the family members present may be reacting out of their internal emotions and thoughts rather than in response to anything particular you have done. The family of a terminally ill cancer patient may be resigned and accepting. They may be grateful for any small kindness you offer. The family of a trauma victim may be angry and aggressive. Recognize that both of these reactions may have little to do with you personally—especially if you are conducting yourself professionally.

Ask

When family members are present, questions must be carefully phrased so that you collect necessary information without raising guilt. In addition to the general history and present illness information you collect, gather information on the patient's religion.

Act

Do whatever is necessary to provide for the patient. You must treat the patient for medical conditions or traumatic injuries as appropriate. If family members are present, it may be comforting for them to know that everything possible is being done. Even simple palliative care, such as placing pillows, may prove very important. Perhaps one of the most important commitments you can make—and make sincerely—is that you, or someone else, will stay by the patient. Even patients who appreciate and accept that they are dying, fear dying alone.

Attend

Listen very carefully to what the patient or the family tells you. This is one of the most important things you can do. You may not be able to honor all their wishes; you have your professional responsibilities. However, you should recognize their concerns and explain why you must do what you do. In most jurisdictions, without written orders to the contrary, EMS providers are required to attempt resuscitation. This may be counter to the wishes of a family with a terminally ill patient at home. Unfortunately, some families do not understand what happens when they call an ambulance and may find themselves in the middle of a scene they did not expect.

Document

In the case presented here, documentation would not pose any special problems, apart from the matter of insurance information. In other cases, it will be necessary to document the decision not to begin resuscitation. There are physical findings that justify a decision not to resuscitate: decay, decapitation, transection, rigor mortis, or dependent lividity. These should be documented carefully. In other cases, there may be a valid **do not resuscitate (DNR) order.** The conditions for validity may vary from state to state. It is important to know your state's policy. Finally, there is the documentation of the patient's physical status.

 CONSIDERATIONS FOR EMS PROVIDERS

First and foremost, recognize that you must not deny your own emotions. Helpers feel anger, rage, disgust, blame, and grief as do families. Share your feelings with others whom you trust. With due regard for confidentiality, let family members know what happened and how you feel. Talk it over with other rescuers and hear how they deal with death. Some will probably show mature, well-considered responses that you can incorporate.

In some cases, such as the death of a child, a friend, or another EMS provider, you may especially benefit from talking through the situation with others. In dealing with the death of a child or coworker, formal debriefings are the best way to start working through your reactions.

If the patient is well known, EMS providers may wish to attend the wake or the funeral. This will not only help them with their grieving process but also may bolster the family as well.

CONCLUSION

Many EMS providers find that their closeness to issues of life and death sets them apart. Sometimes friends and relatives cannot understand your feelings. Those who do not work in close proximity to death can feel uncomfortable around those who do.

REVIEW QUESTIONS

1. What are the five stages in grieving identified by Kübler-Ross?
2. How might a family respond emotionally to the death of a chronically ill member?

3. How might a family respond emotionally to the death of a patient while being transported?

4. When do EMS providers need outside support to help in dealing with death?

EXERCISES

1. Invite a member of the clergy or a hospital chaplain to address your group.

2. Have a group discussion about the deaths EMS providers have witnessed and then review the impact of those events on the families and the EMS providers.

3. Have a near-death survivor address your group.

4. Discuss how the death of person with a chronic illness affects people and EMS providers differently than the death of a healthy child.

5. Discuss the laws governing CPR in your community.

6. Discuss how a family might respond to the death of a chronically ill family member. How might this differ from a family's response to the death of a healthy child?

REFERENCES

1. Martin, L. (1984). *Breathe easy: a guide to lung and respiratory diseases for patients and their families* (p. 34). Englewood Cliffs, NJ: Prentice Hall.

2. Kübler-Ross, E. (1970). *On death and dying.* New York: Macmillan.

3. Thomsen, J. M. (1987). A provider's trauma. *Journal of Emergency Medical Services, 12* (7), 34–37, 40.

FURTHER INFORMATION

Internet Resources

An unusual site for finding out about death and to figure out your life expectancy by using its format: http://www.deathclock.com/

An interesting site offering support in loss: http://www.death-dying.com/

GriefNet.org is an Internet community of people dealing with grief, death, and major loss: http://griefnet.org/

Grief and Children—put out by the American Academy of Child & Adolescent Psychiatry: www.aacap.org/publications/factsfam/grief.htm

Media Resources

Movies

All That Jazz

Steel Magnolias

Ordinary People

Tender Mercies

Terms of Endearment

What's Eating Gilbert Grape

On Your Own Terms Bill Moyers' PBS series

Books

Albom, M. (1997). *Tuesdays with Morrie.* New York: Doubleday.

Kushner, H. (1997). *When bad things happen to good people.* New York: Avon.

Terkel, S. (2001). *Will the circle be unbroken.* New York: New Press.

CHAPTER 15

Multiple Casualty Incident
The Demands, Destruction, and Disorientation

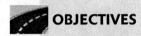

OBJECTIVES

Upon completion of this chapter, you should be able to:

- Explain the physical, psychological, and spiritual challenges of multiple casualty incident (MCI) response.
- Understand the importance of MCI preparedness.
- Describe the role of EMS in mass casualty situations.
- Explain the importance of teamwork.
- Understand the importance of postresponse debriefings.

THE CHALLENGE

A **multiple casualty incident (MCI)**—an incident in which patient needs exceed EMS system resources—creates some of the most demanding conditions you are likely to face. Such an incident is technically demanding, but, more than this, it is physically, psychologically, and spiritually demanding. Even rescuers who are comfortable with everyday emergency work can be overwhelmed by the scope and scale of needs expressed by the victims involved in an MCI.

First, an MCI may be physically demanding either because of difficulties in reaching patients or difficulty of extricating patients who are trapped. However, even when patient access is not a problem, an MCI can be physically demanding because you may make multiple runs between the scene and the hospitals.

Second, an MCI, especially if it involves widespread destruction of property or large numbers of victims, is psychologically disturbing. Rescuers and survivors can be overwhelmed and disoriented by destruction on a large scale. Familiar shapes and landmarks may be disfigured beyond recognition.

Third, an MCI is spiritually disorienting. The sheer magnitude of senseless, sudden injury and death can arouse basic anxieties. Rescuers can be overwhelmed by a deep sense of the fragility of life and even brought to question basic beliefs. Anxiety reactions may not register immediately because your obligation to help is so strong. However, they may remain in your unconscious to emerge as unwanted memories long after the event.

Experience shows that rescuers can get beyond disaster to new levels of awareness and appreciation of life, but it cannot be done alone. In fact, going it alone is a prescription for trouble. The first challenge is to perform one's role as required. The second is to accept one's performance. The third and most difficult challenge is to accept what one has seen and felt and thought and to return to the world of others who have never seen and felt and thought such things.

 ## THE PATIENTS AND THE SITUATION

The fog came in suddenly. Visibility on I-95 dropped to less than 5 feet. Such pea soup fogs were common along the coast in the summer, but rarely did they affect the interstate like this. The cars ahead disappeared. The only guide was

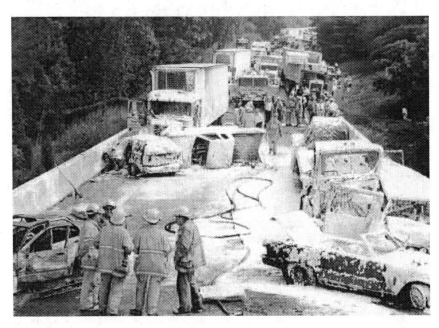

(Courtesy of Baltimore County Fire Department)

the white lane lines. Motorists slowed but not quickly enough. A pickup truck plowed into a station wagon carrying a family on vacation. An eighteen-wheeler jackknifed to avoid colliding with those vehicles. It blocked all three lanes. Two cars collided with the trailer truck. When the chain reaction was over, 25 vehicles were involved. No one on scene could judge the extent or the severity of the incident. The driver of the jackknifed trailer radioed to the state police. He knew that the crash involved at least 10 vehicles, and probably more. He knew there were serious personal injuries but did not know how many.

The state police dispatcher who received the call needed more information than the truck driver could provide. The trucker knew he was southbound but could only describe an approximate location. The dispatcher alerted the police cruiser in the area to investigate. He called for ambulances on standby from five communities along that part of I-95 but could do nothing until he had a better description of the location.

In surveying the wreckage, the trucker realized his first estimate was grossly wrong. He updated the report, stating that, "There are at least 50 cars involved. I can't see 'em all, but I hear people screaming everywhere. For God's sake, get help!" This second estimate was, it turned out, as wrong as the first, but in the opposite direction. It would be several hours before the actual extent of the crash was known.

One of the walking wounded who had emerged from his car was killed when he was hit by a vehicle entering the fog.

A salesman whose car had been hit on the passenger side stood looking feverishly through the trunk of his car for his briefcase.

A state trooper arrived first, coming down the other side of the divided highway. He was able to confirm the multiple vehicle crash and pinpoint the location for other rescue crews, but in the fog he could not assess the extent of the damage or the number of victims. Perhaps more important, he could not cross the highway divider to position his vehicle as a warning to the other rescue vehicles that would be arriving. That responsibility was left for the next arriving cruiser heading southbound.

Mark Wheaton and Steve Mancini were the first ambulance crew to arrive. Their service had been participating in the development of a coordinated **incident command system (ICS)**, but the system had not been finalized. They knew, from the police officers on scene, that other ambulances had been called. In their ambulance they carried a folder with triage tags, but they did not have the complete "first-in" kit, which would contain identifying vests and scene management materials. As the senior medical responder, Mark assumed EMS control and advised the police that he would work closely with them. Steve would be in charge of triage. They established radio contact with the three closest hospitals.

The driver of the station wagon was a woman in her thirties. Her head had hit the windshield. She had not been wearing a seat belt and since she drove an older vehicle there was no air bag. She was bleeding profusely from her left temple. Two children in the car had gotten out. Two others were screaming wildly. One child sat mute, still wondering why his mother did not move.

The driver of the Ford pickup truck was attempting to free his wife, but the passenger-side door had jammed shut.

The lone occupant of a new Lincoln, Ralph Wetherbee, was slumped over the wheel. He did not call for help. He was in cardiac arrest.

A number of drivers and passengers were wandering about. The driver of the pickup enlisted one unharmed man to help him extricate his wife. The truck driver who had originally radioed the police assisted the EMS providers in the area where the least seriously injured were being managed. He made sure that they did not wander out of the triage area.

A radio played on, somewhere in the fog.

The state police, EMS providers, and firefighters jointly assumed incident command. The highway was shut down between the exits of the crash scene, allowing rescue vehicles to approach from either direction.

Mark, Steve, and the other EMS providers who were attempting to treat victims had to make difficult decisions in the first minutes. Ralph Wetherbee was tagged with a black tag and left in his car. The pedestrian who was struck was also marked with a black tag. The wife of the pickup truck driver and the mother in the station wagon were triaged for rapid transport.

It took 5 hours to clear the scene. Besides the two fatalities, 15 patients were transported by ambulance. Another 20 "walking wounded" were transported by school bus.

The "killer fog" was reported in the news media throughout the state. The national television networks also picked up dramatic pictures of the wreckage, clearly visible when the fog had cleared.

In the wake of the disaster, the responding rescue workers and police were given commendations by the governor. Some of those commended did not feel comfortable with what they had done.

Several weeks later, while transporting a stable patient down that same stretch of I-95, Steve Mancini turned to Mark Wheaton and said, "I can't get that scene out of my mind." After a short pause, Mark agreed, "Neither can I. You just can't get used to something like that."

 THE PATIENTS' WORLDS

An MCI not only strains the resources of the emergency system; it strains the coping abilities of victims. Remember that the victims of MCIs are typically normal individuals who are temporarily stressed. Their world does not include disaster, and they have not worked through appropriate roles for the calamitous situation.

There are seven distinct stages to a disaster or mass casualty situation: warning, threat, impact, inventory, rescue, remedy, and recovery (see Box 15–1).[1] In a hurricane, there may be substantial time for many of those who will be affected to prepare. In events such as a killer fog or earthquake, there may be little or no warning or sense of threat. Where there is some time to gather up possessions or to take precautions to prevent some damage or injuries, victims may be somewhat better prepared. However, for those who must respond, the period of warning or threat can be an anxious time. Rescuers must prepare themselves and their families and must make the basic decisions concerning their responsibilities. The impact phase will also differ in different types of MCIs. Large-scale disasters will affect whole communities, and even some of those not immediately physically injured will suffer significant psychological consequences.[2]

As an EMS provider, you will usually be concerned with immediate reactions. However, it is important to consider later effects also. During remedy and recovery periods, there will still be emergency needs to be met: some will be delayed effects of the MCI itself; others will be related to the remedy and recovery operations; still others will be the "normal" emergency service needs of the community. These periods pose their own difficulties both for the survivors and the rescuers, who may be physically and mentally exhausted.

Whether disaster strikes without warning or with an intensity for which victims did not have a chance to prepare, it thrusts patients into a world in which orienting landmarks have been destroyed or disappeared and in which disfigurement and death abruptly replace the normal expectations of everyday life.[3] Patients must make major adjustments without warning or forethought. Similar immediate reactions also occur in bystanders and rescuers.[4]

The disaster has mental consequences as well as physical ones that extend over a long period of time. Anxiety, depression, post-traumatic disorders, and

---

BOX 15–1

SEVEN STAGES IN A DISASTER SITUATION

1. Warning
2. Threat
3. Impact
4. Inventory
5. Rescue
6. Remedy
7. Recovery

constrained emotional range are common. Through flashbacks, intrusive images, and nightmares, patients can continue to experience the catastrophic event.[5]

 THE BEHAVIOR OF THE PATIENTS

During the warning or threat phase, some potential victims will experience panic and anxiety reactions, which can cause problems for the emergency response system itself. Perhaps the most dramatic example of such behavior is the famous "War of the Worlds" broadcast of 1938. The story began with a realistic news report that Earth was being invaded by Martians. Many people believed the story and reacted as if it were true. During the actual impact phase, patients may respond in a variety of ways. Some will panic, running aimlessly about or, if trapped, screaming and flailing about. Such panic is often contagious. Others will wander about purposelessly. This response may be psychological, but it may also be a result of injury, especially head injury. Others become paralyzed with anxiety. They remain passive, mute, inactive. Being involved in a multiple casualty situation takes a great deal of energy, especially if the victim has sought to escape. By the time rescuers arrive, the victims may be physically exhausted even if they are unharmed.[2]

 THE EMOTIONS AND THOUGHTS BEHIND THE BEHAVIOR

People caught in a multiple casualty situation show a wide range of emotions. Two of the most common are apparent opposites: unrestricted emotional release and emotional shutdown. The panicked victim is flooded by emotion. The numbed victim effectively shuts down all emotions. This shutdown may be associated with the psychological defense of denial.

Thinking processes are also radically changed. Most victims are disoriented: they have lost their familiar landmarks. In our scenario, the fog was significantly disorienting; in other cases a person might be absorbed by the enormity of a storm, ignoring the suffering all around; but even when there is no external reason for disorientation, psychological disorientation is normal. For some, disorientation may take the form of preoccupation with the fate of loved ones and the denial of their own injuries. For others, disorientation may take the form of an overwhelming concern with the victim's personal responsibility for the disaster. "If only I'd stopped; if I hadn't been traveling so fast; if I hadn't been so close." For others, the disaster situation will have brought the patient face to face with his or her own mortality. Many will turn to prayer.[6]

The disaster continues to affect patients' and rescuers' behaviors, thoughts, and emotions long after the immediate threat has passed. A significant later effect is survivor guilt. It is important to recognize these effects. We will discuss these effects on EMS providers in Chapter 16 and things they can do to deal with them in Chapter 17.

 FAMILY/BYSTANDER RESPONSES

Those who observe the disaster and those whose loved ones are caught up in it often experience similar reactions to those physically injured in the event.

Some detach themselves by focusing on a particular detail and ignoring the larger situation. For example, the salesman blotted out the destruction around him by focusing on his missing briefcase filled with important documents. Others become involved as organizers and rescuers, some being highly effective and others confusing rescue efforts. The truck driver, for example, was helpful in keeping the least seriously injured patients within the triage area.

This variety of behaviors found among the noninjured or minimally injured reflects an important point: the behavior of survivors of a disaster often serves to protect them psychologically. Some behavior will be helpful; other behavior gets in the way or complicates rescue. Do not assume that a helpful victim will not need psychological help after the fact.

 PROVIDER RESPONSES

Events that stress the EMS system beyond its capacity to provide adequate care for all patients will affect EMS providers. Dr. Joseph Waeckerle, an emergency physician who was instrumental in the rescue operations at the Kansas City Hyatt hotel disaster, speaking to emergency physicians, estimated that "only 10% to 20% [of you] . . . will be able to walk into a disaster site and effectively collect your thoughts, get yourself together, and be able to function objectively and professionally for the next 12, 24, or 36 hours."[7] EMS providers and others also face special problems not faced by bystanders: they will feel accountable for the success or failure of their efforts.

Many EMS providers will never be called to respond to an MCI; however, the potential is there. In some cases, the environment contains hazards or potential hazards that services can and should train for specifically. For example, areas with geological faults are at high risk for earthquakes; other areas have known flood, hurricane, or tornado risks. More specifically, some manufacturing plants will present hazards that must be understood and planned for by all agencies that have a responsibility to respond.

The terrorist attacks of September 11, 2001 raised many new concerns for emergency personnel. While for most EMS providers the likelihood of responding to terrorist violence is less than that of responding to a multiple vehicle crash, these concerns must be included in training and preparation.

INTERVENTION STRATEGIES

Every community and every service should have incident command structures for MCI responses, and every ambulance service should have policies and procedures that support this structure. It is important to train and test these plans through regular drills.

Observe

Your safety is a primary concern. If you are not appropriately cross-trained, you must follow ambulance policies and procedures about entering hazardous situations and know your limitations. If you are injured in the line of duty, you will help no one. The first EMS providers on the scene have a special obligation to observe, not only for hazards, but also to provide more accurate information to dispatchers and other arriving units.

Interact

Unlike most other scenes, the opportunity for interaction will be considerably limited. The greatest good of the greatest number of patients requires limited personal interactions and personal reassurance. However, interaction is still important. In fact, one of the most important things that you can do is convey a sense of control. Many victims will draw strength from the sense of control they see in the rescuers. However, if the rescuers are themselves unsure, victims will quickly pick this up. As the scene becomes more organized, it is possible that many of the less severely hurt can help in providing minor first aid to other victims whose treatment is not high priority.

Television, radio, and newspaper reporters will probably be among the first on the scene. Your service should have policies for cooperating with incident command to handle press inquiries. Follow them.

Ask

Because opportunities for interaction are limited and triage and treatment protocols must be followed, your first questions will be important in quickly establishing that the patient's airway is patent and whether or not he or she is alert and oriented.

Act

Triage decision making demands the greatest good for the greatest number. This means bypassing patients in cardiac arrest or patients whose injuries are so devastating that they are unlikely to survive. Further, "preserving life takes precedence over preservation of limbs."[8] These rules are sound, but applying them involves you in a potentially stressful decision-making process. Anxiety over correctness of triage decisions may recur with news reports and media interviews with survivors or with the relatives of the deceased.

Attend

It is not possible to listen as you would in other situations or to attend any one patient for too long. However, you can enlist others so that those patients on delayed transport status will not feel abandoned.

Document

Documentation and debriefing are important in the follow-up to any multiple casualty situation. This is one of the areas in EMS in which more effective techniques of scene control and management are being constantly developed. Documentation and case review will help to improve the care offered in other MCIs.

 ## CONSIDERATIONS FOR EMS PROVIDERS

While the best laid plans may fail to work out completely, planning and education are essential if EMS providers and others are to perform at their best in a mass casualty situation. First, if there is a state or regional ICS in place, all EMS providers must understand it and their roles. If there is no systemwide ICS, the service must have appropriate policies and procedures worked out in advance with other responding agencies.

EMS providers should be clear beforehand on what their employer expects of them. Dodson[9] presents these as a series of questions. Some of these are relevant to our concerns:

"What about my family and loved ones? I have a duty to them also!"

"Since the roads are closed to routine traffic, can I drive past the house and school in the unit to check on them?"

"Who will care for my children if I am held at work?"

"I may need to take my elderly parents to an evacuation center in an unaffected area. Will I be excused?"

Following an MCI, EMS providers themselves may experience significant stress-related physical responses including nausea, vomiting, diarrhea, muscle tremors, agitation, fatigue, restlessness, insomnia, moodiness, and difficulty in concentrating.[1] Even if overt physical signs and symptoms are absent, the effects can take an emotional toll if they are not dealt with appropriately. Often responders will have problems in relationships after being involved in an MCI.

We believe very strongly in critical incident stress debriefing (CISD) for EMS providers and others. This is a separate process from incident critique. In fact, in contrast to the formal critique, CISD results are limited to those specifically involved in the rescue operations.[10] Similar programs are also useful for the husbands and wives and older children of rescuers who have been exposed to stresses in the line of duty.

CONCLUSION

Because an MCI stresses the system, it stresses those who are on the front lines. Triage decisions, concern for family and colleagues, and fatigue from long hours of scene work can take their toll. These incidents test skill and character, but you will make a decisive difference.

REVIEW QUESTIONS

1. What are the seven stages of a disaster?
2. What are some of the ways in which patients respond to a multiple casualty incident?
3. What types of concerns will EMS providers have when responding to a disaster?
4. How should an ambulance service prepare for a multiple casualty incident?
5. What are some of the delayed psychological effects of a disaster on the participants?

EXERCISES

1. Watch one of Hollywood's disaster movies, then discuss how accurate it is.
2. What would you do if you were in the middle of a disaster?
3. Have a disaster survivor review and discuss the ordeal.

REFERENCES

1. Hafen, B., & Frandsen, K. (1986). *Psychological emergencies and crisis intervention*. Englewood, CO: Morton Publishing.
2. Erikson, K. T. (1976). *Everything in its path: destruction of community in the Buffalo Creek flood*. New York: Simon & Schuster.
3. Lifton, R. J., & Olson, E. (1986). The meaning of human disaster. In R. H. Moos (Ed.). *Coping with life crises: an integrated approach* (p. 301). New York: Plenum Press.

4. http://www.angelfire.com/sys/popup_source.shtml?search_string=julian + ford/2002

5. www.fema.gov/2002

6. http://www.mentalhealth.org/emhs/emergencyservices/2002

7. Nordberg, M. (1990). When disaster strikes. *Journal of Emergency Medical Services, 19* (6), 42–43, 45, 48–50.

8. Hubble, M. W., & Hubble, S. D. (2001). *Principles of advanced trauma care.* Clifton Park, NY: Delmar Learning.

9. Dodson, D. (1987). Catastrophe! Questions paramedics should ask their supervisors. *Journal of Emergency Medical Services, 12* (9), 44–49.

10. Mitchell, J. T., & Bray, G. (1990). *Emergency services stress.* Englewood Cliffs, NJ: Brady Communications.

FURTHER INFORMATION

Internet Resources

American College of Surgeons: www.facs.org

American College of Emergency Physicians: www.acep.org

EMS Bulletin *All Providers Need Mass Casualty Incident Management Training* (Winter 2000). Module I should be taught in EMS courses and as continuing education for EMS providers. The module includes basic first steps every EMS provider should know: www.vdh.state.va.us/oems/b14wi0014.htm

Federal Emergency Management Agency: www.fema.gov/fema

Federal Emergency Management Agency FACT SHEET DISASTER ASSISTANCE PROGRAMS. Various disaster assistance programs are available under a presidential disaster declaration: www.jeffcomo.org/fema.html

Homeland Defense Weapons of Mass Destruction (WMD) Installation Preparedness (IP) Courses Fact Sheet: www.2.sbccom.army.mil/hld/ip/fs/wmd_ip_courses_fact_sheet.htm

Media Resources

Movies

Escape from New York

MASH

The Sum of All Fears

CHAPTER 16

Street and System Stresses

Recognition Is the Key

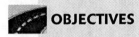
OBJECTIVES

Upon completion of this chapter, you should be able to:

■ Explain the major sources of stress for EMS providers.

■ Describe how different stress management techniques might help at different times.

■ Demonstrate effective teamwork in helping stressed colleagues.

THE CHALLENGE

The satisfactions of being an EMS provider are great: knowing how to save lives and reduce pain, and having the opportunity to truly make a difference. However, there are few other jobs in which workers are exposed to as much suffering, despair, and plain human folly as in emergency medical service. Your experiences will affect you and your family. Sometimes these effects build up so gradually that you do not see the subtle changes that occur in yourself and your colleagues. Keeping up the self-confidence essential to respond effectively on the streets can lead to an inflated sense of self-importance and an inability to realistically appraise one's weaknesses. Relaxing after work with other EMS providers at the bar can be an important outlet for tension and anger, yet it can lead to use of alcohol as self-medication to deaden pain. Seeing the humor in the human condition can help to ease your pain, but it can also become heart-hardening when patients are demeaned and stereotyped. Work stresses can carry over into home life, poisoning family relationships.

This chapter looks at some of your stresses and suggests constructive ways to deal with them. As Bray[1] suggests, it is necessary to recognize the potential for significant problems well before a critical incident or the accumulation of stresses results in a personal crisis. One of the challenges you face as an EMS provider is to grow through your care of others in order to provide even better care for those whom you serve.

 THE SITUATION

A group of EMS providers have come together at lunch at the state EMS conference. They compare notes on the educational sessions they have attended and begin to swap "war stories." Paul Appleton tells the story of "Mr. Lime Green," who is well known for his bizarre taste in socks and who seems to need an ambulance every time Paul is on duty. Mike Devereaux says he'd rather deal with body odors than with AIDS and hepatitis B. Helen Johnson, a rural volunteer, remarks that, "At least in the big city, you've got some solid management support and can look out for each other better than we volunteers can." "Yeah, sure!" John Paulson says, "My boss is a loud-mouthed SOB who cares more about the insurance form than patient care. I get a load of crap if I come back without an insurance number. I know guys who don't even do an assessment, but they'll get that number. That's what counts with my boss." "Don't think that third service EMS is any better," says Betty James. "The command staff is so caught up in making themselves look good for the commissioner that they'll sweep a lot of dirt under the rug."

Paul Appleton looks at his watch. It is time to move on to the next session. Paul thinks about the sometimes sharp contrasts between the picture of EMS

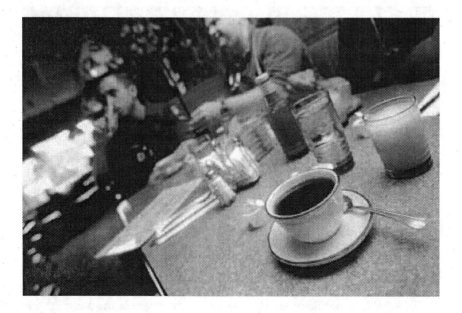

presented in some of the lectures and the one that emerges in casual conversations during lunch.

 ## THE EMS PROVIDER'S WORLD

It is important to recognize that you work in a world of "betweens." In one sense, you are a go-between. Work places you between the family and the patient, between the patient and the hospital, between the community and the hospital, between life and death.[2–4] In another sense you experience wild swings in the nature of work. In the course of a shift, you can go between extremes of boredom and business, and between burning with enthusiasm and burning out. All the betweens create stress. And the stress affects you and your family.

 ## THE EMS PROVIDER'S BEHAVIOR

Normally, we expect EMS providers to work professionally and responsibly with a sense of their own limits. In general, these responsibilities should be spelled out in an organizational mission statement that is consistent with training and licensure requirements.

Stress can arise from many sources. Some are job related, such as the stress of patient care or the stress of managing shift work. Others are not: stressful family relationships, economic concerns, health concerns. Stress can lead to two very different behavioral responses. The first of these is withdrawal. Withdrawing EMS providers become isolated from coworkers, family, and friends. This type of behavior is popularly associated with burnout. They do the minimum, take all their breaks, and rarely volunteer. They call in sick frequently. In general, they are "there, but not there." Withdrawal may also be associated with alcohol and other drug use.[5] Drugs can offer a means of blotting out painful experiences and job pressures. Drugs such as alcohol can be addictive, and an alcoholic will lose control over the ability to limit use of the drug and will need greater and greater amounts to provide the same degree of relief.

The second type of behavior is overinvolvement. In response to stress, an EMS provider may become a workaholic, a "super-EMS provider." A super-EMS provider is always around the station; he or she cannot get enough of EMS, frequently volunteers, takes all the education classes offered, and often becomes an instructor. In general, the super-EMS providers are always there. The problem is that work assumes a disproportionate importance in life. Needing to be in control becomes a consuming passion. Family and friends and other interests may be neglected.

Stress also shows up in disorders of daily living. Some EMS providers experience a loss of appetite; others find themselves eating to excess or bingeing.

Some develop insomnia; others sleep too much. Some lose all interest in sex; others have a heightened sex drive. Some have nightmares about what they have seen and heard; others have daydreams about saving lives.

THE EMOTIONS AND THOUGHTS BEHIND THE BEHAVIOR

Work affects feelings and thoughts, and feelings and thoughts affect work. When a patient dies in the ambulance or when you treat a small child whom you believe to be a victim of abuse, you are disturbed by the situation. When a run goes well or when a man with a myocardial infarction (MI) is safely and comfortably brought to the hospital, you are elated. The feelings can be brief, but these momentary feelings, good or bad, may lead to more lasting feelings that color the way you see the world.

If feelings are not accepted and worked through, EMS providers may develop dysfunctional responses. We note four of these here. The first three are generally associated with burnout, the fourth with a workaholic reaction.

First, some EMS providers develop a sense of persistent sadness or melancholy. Images of patients who "died on their watch," memories of battered women and children, and recollections of the chronically ill and the dying may lead to pessimism and fatalism; at worst, these unresolved experiences may lead to clinical depression.

Second, EMS providers may develop chronic anxiety. Tense and irritable, an anxious EMS provider dreads the next dispatch or the next run, always anticipating the worst.

Third, EMS providers may become indifferent and distant. Sometimes this distance from patients shows up in inappropriate gallows humor or in a tendency to stereotype patients and bystanders.

Fourth, EMS providers may actually feel "high" on the action of emergency response and become too enthusiastic. This behavior may be accompanied by an overemphasis on the technical side of care.

Stress affects thought and the thinking process.[6] For some EMS providers, painful, distressing images can come to dominate their lives. An EMS provider may not be able to help recalling an incident marked by senseless suffering or loss, or an incident in which he or she felt helpless or conflicted, such as might occur when called on to respond to a fire scene or to a hazardous material (HAZMAT) incident in which the EMS provider is not trained to effect a rescue. In such instances, guilt can be a powerful source of stress. The EMS provider who lost the patient with chronic obstructive pulmonary disease (COPD) on the way to a scheduled hospital visit wonders if she could have done more. In other cases, an EMS provider may experience survivor guilt. For example, one crew could not respond to an emergency because of engine trouble; another crew was sent. On the way to the scene the ambulance collided head on with another vehicle. The driver died. The crew that did not respond was marked by survivor guilt. Less devastating, but also important forms of survivor guilt occur when crew members are laid off.

Flashbacks can be quite common. An EMS provider may suddenly relive a traumatic event. Quite often a flashback can be triggered by some stimulus that seems completely neutral to others: a song on the radio, a smell, a conversational reference. Sometimes a natural condition such as fog or black ice may trigger a flashback.

When the conscious mind represses or denies an unpleasant event, a trauma may come to the surface in disturbing dream images. The unconscious continues to rework and attempt to come to grips with the devastation that the conscious mind has denied. For example, one crew member caught up in the carnage from a multiple casualty incident (MCI) feared the night because, "bodies haunt my sleep."

Despite the fact that we can identify common stressors in emergency work, what stresses one EMS provider may not stress another, or a minor irritant for one EMS provider may be a major stressor for another. Well-meaning but casual advice to "chill out" may leave a stressed EMS provider feeling isolated and misunderstood. The stress a person feels is a result of

- The event
- Personal perceptions of the event
- Personal dynamics

Therefore, it is important to remember that what constitutes a major stress for one EMS provider may not be stressful for another.

Sometimes EMS providers forget that they take for granted a level of violence and pain that others would find overwhelming. Not even emergency department (ED) staff in a trauma center have to deal with the same level of carnage as the EMS providers who have to work with the tangled steel and raw injuries at the scene.[7] Even in situations that do not involve blood and feces, the EMS provider often must deal with raw emotions that patients and families have not had time to process.

Each EMS provider brings specific expectations to each scene. Prior to arriving at a scene, an EMS provider has formed some expectations based on past experiences. If these past experiences have been largely successful, then he or she may feel less stressed. However, a situation that has been painful or difficult in the past can trigger anxiety and stress.

Each EMS provider also brings a personal history that is unrelated to past EMS experience. Some EMS providers will be more comfortable with ambiguity than others. An EMS provider who is uncomfortable with ambiguity may have more difficulty dealing with a medical patient with complex symptoms or with a psychiatric emergency patient than with a trauma patient in hypovolemic shock.

Sometimes patient characteristics can trigger stress reactions. A patient who reminds an EMS provider of a mother or father or wife or daughter can trigger stress reactions that seem totally out of place to other EMS providers.

Finally, there is stress that follows from the EMS provider's need to adjust to variable work schedules and activity patterns. Some EMS providers will have no problem adapting to 24-hour shifts or to 10-hour/14-hour patterns; others will find such alterations disruptive. Some EMS providers will find that the pattern of long stretches of routine punctuated by high levels of activity is an exciting way to work; others will prefer more structured activity patterns. Finally, there is the stress of facing potentially life-threatening situations. While most EMS providers do not face threats of physical violence in everyday work, they do face the threat of contact with infectious disease and the challenge of driving under emergency conditions.

Before moving on to consider treatment of stress, it is important to point out that stress is not necessarily a bad thing. Stress is necessary to promote personal growth and change. Everyone has an ideal level of stress stimulation. If the amount of stress exceeds this level, the individual feels overwhelmed. Too little stress results in feelings of chronic boredom.

 ## FAMILY/WORKPLACE RESPONSES

Patient-related incidents are not the only stressors in the life of an EMS provider. Conflicts between family relationships and responsibilities and in work relationships can produce significant stresses.

There are two different kinds of demands that place burdens on an EMS provider's family. First, EMS is psychologically demanding. Family members may not understand or appreciate the depth of importance of an EMS provider's commitment. Quite often a family will not be able to relate to the EMS provider's work, creating a chasm that is difficult to bridge. However, they may not understand the EMS provider's inability (for professional or for personal reasons) to share some of the troubling things that happen at work. Second, EMS providers who work unusual shifts are often stressed by difficulties in managing family and work responsibilities. Working 12- or 24-hour shifts disrupts the flow of family life.

Many ambulance services have serious financial or management problems. These problems may create anxiety that affects patient care and employee health as well. Organizational politics can be a major source of stress. When cooperative relationships between management and workers or between coworkers break down, they often move through three stages: open conflict, domination–subordination, and isolation. Being involved in any one of these three types of relationships[8] generates substantial stresses over and above the stress of patient care. Under conditions of conflict, workers are hypervigilant.

They constantly scan their environment anticipating trouble. In one service, following several rapid changes in management and a brutal budget cut, the crews found themselves constantly on guard.

Domination–subordination can follow if conflicts cannot be satisfactorily resolved. The "losing side" may fall back to "working to rule," or doing the minimum possible. Memoranda replace face-to-face communication.

Finally, a relationship can deteriorate to the point that communication among managers and workers or between workers stops. Under these circumstances patient care and employee health will certainly suffer.

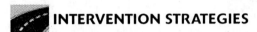 ## INTERVENTION STRATEGIES

Stress cannot only be described and explained, it can—and must—be managed.[1,7–9] In the following sections we discuss three general considerations: the necessity of (1) early recognition, (2) timing of responses, and (3) different strategies. Then we turn to some specific strategies that others have found helpful.

Recognition

Before you can deal with a stressor, you must recognize it.[1,10] As obvious as this may sound, quite often people deny sources of stress in their lives or rationalize them away with statements such as "that's just the way things have to be." For instance, an EMS provider may be so driven to help that he or she suppresses or denies the psychic toll that interrupted sleep is taking. A person who has always worked in a poorly managed organization can come to take poor management for granted, blaming it on external causes—the government, the reimbursement system—beyond the control of management.

An individual can come to recognize stress in a number of ways. Many will come to recognize it on their own. Others will not identify stress with reaction to a particular incident but rather will recognize that they are overstressed when they are "sick and tired of feeling sick and tired." For those who are close to awareness, a leader's gentle suggestion that others who have been through what your crew has been through can be severely stressed may be all that is needed to bring stress to consciousness. The crew that returned from the disaster in the fog merely needed the chief's statement that "It must've been hell out there" to unburden themselves. For those still unable to recognize the effects of stress, an outside expert may be necessary.

However, the best "cure" is prevention. It is unfortunate that, although stress is widely recognized as a factor in the life of many EMS providers, it has not been given its due in the training curricula. Such attention would underscore not only the need for recognition but would also alert EMS providers to the methods available for dealing with stress. Articles in EMS journals can provide a general understanding that others have felt the same way. Many an EMS provider, who might feel isolated in his or her own squad, has been comforted by the written accounts of other EMS providers who have felt stress, anxiety, or depression as a result of their work.

Timing

Effective response to stress is essential. The critical incident stress debriefing (CISD) literature demonstrates the importance of rapidly addressing EMS providers' concerns following a traumatic incident.[11,12] However, stress cannot always be dealt with immediately. The crews returning from the disaster in the fog were physically exhausted and needed to be there for their own families who were worried about their safety.

In other situations in which stress is organizational, rather than incident related, restoring cooperative relationships and an atmosphere of trust may take considerable time, but it is necessary for one party to make the first move. This can be threatening, but generally the threat is lessened if one states clearly at the outset that he or she is feeling stressed, separating the feeling from the personalities involved. Fisher and Ury's excellent book *Getting to Yes*[13] provides excellent guidance for principled negotiation. Usually, when organizational issues are predominant, the best time to talk about stressors is when both parties are willing to talk. It can be counterproductive for one side to impose a specific meeting time on the other.

Intervention

No one intervention strategy works for all.[14] Just as volunteer units may have different satisfactions and stresses than career services and each may be different from private services, no one approach to stress intervention will work for all services.[15] This idea may seem obvious, but too often when squad members feel overwhelmed, they look for an immediate, simple solution. For example, after a conference, EMS providers may come back with "the answer." For the next several weeks they may test the patience of everyone else in the service until they realize that they have found an answer, not *the* answer.

Despite the fact that no one intervention will suit all situations, there is one approach that is clearly wrong: failing to explore and resolve stressful issues will hurt individuals and squads in the long run.[1,10] Unresolved emotions and unexplored ideas hamper individual effectiveness and cooperation.

In psychological crisis situations, decisive intervention is required. An EMS provider who is drinking or taking drugs on duty, or whose work performance is impaired because of alcohol or other drug abuse, needs firm and well-coordinated treatment. An EMS provider experiencing clinical depression or other major psychological disturbance needs more help than can be provided by well-meaning colleagues. A well-designed employee assistance program (EAP) should be able to guide such troubled individuals to the appropriate treatments.

SPECIFIC INTERVENTION METHODS

In considering interventions, we focus on prevention strategies, early-intervention strategies, and later-intervention strategies. Prevention strategies include developing a mission statement, practicing health maintenance, balancing life interests, and education. In addition, managers can be effective stress-prevention agents.

Prevention

Develop a "Mission Statement." The best stress management approach is to develop conditions in which you can reach the maximum of your potential within the opportunities at hand. This approach is as important in families and social groups as it is in work groups, but it is often neglected in all these types of settings. As Stephen Covey says in *Seven Habits of Highly Effective People*, this is a continuing process that begins with being proactive, or taking initiative, rather than being acted on.[16]

EMS providers tend to find themselves in two very different types of circumstances that can lead to stress: chronic overstimulation or chronic understimulation. A proactive approach will prevent either of these two circumstances from developing or will seek to address overstimulating or understimulating situations early on. An organizational and personal mission statement that defines appropriate responsibilities and limits will help you to focus and to prevent imbalance.

Practice Health Maintenance. Unhealthy lifestyles lead to, and exacerbate the effects of, stress. Being overweight, self-medicating with alcohol or other drugs, lack of exercise, and lack of rest can compound the effects of stress at work. A regular physical examination by a physician who understands the demands of EMS and who can identify appropriate physical exercise and diet is invaluable.

Balance Life Interests and Activities. Stress develops when life interests are out of balance. There are two different types of balance that are important. The first is the balance among personal time, family time, and work time. The second is the balance among physical, mental, and spiritual development. Because most EMS involves work in 24-hour-a-day organizations and because most EMS providers work irregular and overtime hours, these balances are difficult to maintain.

Educate Yourself. Education is important in stress management in three different ways. First, a well-educated EMS provider will have a greater repertoire of technical skills and a greater level of comfort in using those skills. He or she will be less likely to become stressed in the field. Second, education will prepare an EMS provider to deal with the many different types of situations that he or she will encounter in the field, to recognize psychological features of patients (and EMS providers), and to maintain a professional attitude in the face of conflict or ingratitude. Third, education that directly teaches breathing exercises, relaxation, meditation, and physical-conditioning methods provides the EMS provider with an increased repertoire of stress-reduction skills.

Encourage Constructive Management Practices. Four management practices can be recommended for any service.[17-19] First, managers must respect the abilities of employees. Employees should be "praised in public, criticized in private." If errors in patient care are to be discussed in a case-review session, these should be discussed with the individuals involved first. Second, management can provide opportunities for appropriate EMS provider participation in decision making. As EMS providers grow with the service, they may appreciate the opportunity to participate in management decisions. EMS providers will certainly benefit from educational programs that assume or acknowledge their experience. Third, management should prepare EMS providers for changes by discussing needs and rationales before implementing or announcing changes officially. Finally, management should set achievable objectives for the service and direct EMS providers toward their accomplishment. If management does not provide this kind of support in a particular situation, it is generally appropriate to suggest such changes for the future.

Early Intervention

Stress can build up gradually, or it can suddenly overwhelm an EMS provider confronted with a personally challenging situation. The prevention measures noted earlier will reduce the magnitude of stress responses but will not completely eliminate dysfunctional stress responses. For example, a generally healthy lifestyle will prepare you for handling physically and emotionally challenging situations. An active spiritual life will provide necessary support for dealing with loss and suffering. Educational programs will prepare you for working with and through some of the most difficult situations you will face. However, the reality of the death of a child or any unexpected death, or the breakdown in communications between partners or between EMS providers and managers, will still present stresses that cannot be anticipated and that cannot be ignored. Some measures can be taken by individuals working in their own best interests; others will require management support.

Early-intervention strategies are strategies that help you to monitor changes in your behavior, thoughts, and emotions. We recommend three practices: keeping a journal, listening to your family, and managing schedules and work loads equitably. In addition, management can play an important role by monitoring relationships within the service and with other professionals.

Individual Early-Intervention Strategies

Keep a Journal. Keeping a journal or a record of your work experiences, needs, and satisfactions can be a powerful tool in releasing anxiety and in monitoring your own fluctuating emotional and physical state. Just a simple log (with due regard for patient confidentiality) can be an important outlet.

Listen to Your Family. Many EMS providers do not know how to involve families effectively. Many non-EMS wives and husbands (and children) are very uncomfortable listening to or talking about disease and trauma. Yet, it is important that they understand how EMS work may affect an EMS provider, and it is also important for an EMS provider to understand why others may not be as fascinated with "war stories" as their colleagues are.

Management Early-Intervention Strategies

Manage Schedules and Work Loads Equitably. Perhaps the single most effective management approach to managing stress is to manage schedules. This task should involve scheduling time to allow individuals to satisfy their needs and develop their potentials and should also include managing partnerships to maximize effective working relationships.

Monitor Relationships Among Workers. People function most effectively in cooperative relationships. When partners or coworkers begin to feel repeated conflicts, engage in power struggles, or withdraw and isolate themselves, stress develops. Early prevention requires self-monitoring and management monitoring to identify conflict situations and to deal with these situations before they degenerate into power struggles or isolation.

Monitor Relationships with Other Professionals. EMS providers also are greatly affected by their relationships with physicians and nurses. A supportive ED is an important ally for the ambulance service. Unfortunately, many nurses and physicians do not appreciate what EMS providers do. They have only slight knowledge of life on the streets and expect EMS providers to have a level of knowledge that exceeds their emergency medical training. Sometimes these misunderstandings can be corrected through case presentations, rounds, or educational programs presented by hospital staff. In other cases, it might be valuable for EMS providers to observe in the ED or for ED personnel to ride along with the ambulance crew.

Later-Intervention Strategies

Later interventions are methods that become necessary when other methods have failed to contain or control stresses. That does not mean that you can ignore these methods until something happens. To be most effective, the structure has to be present well before the later-intervention services are needed. Three of these are especially important: critical incident stress debriefing (CISD), employee assistance, and availability of individual therapy opportunities.

Critical Incident Stress Debriefing. CISD should be an integral part of every service. We have already discussed the importance of having CISD programs set up before one is needed. Events such as an incident that results in the death of a child, a multiple casualty incident (MCI), or a response in which other rescuers are seriously injured or killed should be followed up with stress debriefing for the rescuers involved. In this process, a team will meet specifically with the personnel involved and discuss the incident. CISD is not therapy, but a debriefing that gives the participants the opportunity to express and work through the normal feelings they have in response to an abnormal situation.

Employee Assistance Referrals. For many EMS providers with work-related problems, employee assistance is the first step toward mastering them.[19] It is important that the program be supported by the employees or the union and that records be confidential. The key factor in determining the need for referral is the effect of a problem on job performance. Further referrals may be justified.

Individual or Group Psychotherapy. Moving into a therapeutic program can be frightening, because many persons with problems cling to their problems rather than face change that can be even more frightening. An organizational support system that encourages employees to seek support before personal problems become job problems is important. It is important to have an insurance program that will cover the costs of psychiatric or psychological treatment.

CONCLUSION

Being an EMS provider is stressful, but it is also rewarding, often in surprising ways. It is not necessarily the big "save" or the heroic rescue that is most memorable. The most memorable event of your career may be the smile of gratitude from an elderly patient whom you have treated considerately, or the time that you were there to hold the hand of a dying cancer patient when nothing more could be done.

Such experiences can bring us closer to the important things in life and give us a perspective and a depth few other people ever have the opportunity to experience.

REVIEW QUESTIONS

1. What are some of the extreme responses that may indicate that an EMS provider is becoming stressed out?

2. What are the four ways in which stress can affect an EMS provider?

3. Is stress always bad?

4. How may job conditions affect family life?

5. What types of stress management techniques fit best with your lifestyle?

EXERCISES

1. List the top 10 stresses you or your group experience on the job.
2. Describe how work stress is carried home.
3. List people's reactions to stress.
4. Discuss which stress management approaches work best for your lifestyle.

REFERENCES

1. Bray, G. (1988). Stress: using the REAPER model to learn to cope. *Journal of Emergency Medical Services, 13* (9), 54–60.
2. Heightman, A. J. (2001). Impact 9-11. *Journal of Emergency Medical Services, 26* (10), 51–52.
3. Maggiore, W. A. (1996). Substance abuse. *Journal of Emergency Medical Services, 21* (11), 66–67, 71–72, 76–78, 80.
4. Roberts, S. W., & Karren, K. J. (1987). Job satisfaction among paramedics. *Journal of Emergency Medical Services, 12* (3), 48–49.
5. Avis, H. (1999). *Drugs and life* (4th ed.). New York: McGraw-Hill.
6. Ward, M. J. (2001). Attack on the Pentagon. *Journal of Emergency Medical Services, 27* (4), 22–24, 26–27, 30, 32, 34.
7. Murphy, P. & Taigman, C. F. (2001). Caring for Karen. *Journal of Emergency Medical Services, 27* (1), 36–38, 40.
8. Huder, R. C. (1987). Burnout: The preventable disease. *Journal of Emergency Medical Services, 12* (3), 50–54.
9. Melton, E. I. (1988). What resuscitation does for the rescuer. *Journal of Emergency Medical Services, 13* (8), 8–11.
10. Soreff, S. (1981). *Management of the psychiatric emergency.* New York: John Wiley & Sons.
11. Mitchell, J. T. (1988). Stress: the history, status and future of critical incident stress debriefings. *Journal of Emergency Medical Services, 13* (11), 46–52.
12. Soreff, S. (1979). Sudden death in the emergency department: a comprehensive approach for families, emergency medical technicians, and emergency department staff. *Critical Care Medicine, 7* (321), 321–323.
13. Fisher, R., & Ury, S. (1991). *Getting to yes.* New York: Penguin Books.
14. Miller, G. T., Gordon, D. L., Issenberg, S. B., La Combe, D. M. & Brotons, A. A. (2001). Teamwork. *Journal of Emergency Medical Services 24* (12), 44–51.

15. Hoeger, W. & Hoeger, S. (1999). *Principles and labs for physical fitness* (2nd ed.). Englewood, CO.: Morton Publishing Company.

16. Covey, S. (1990). *Seven habits of highly effective people.* New York: Simon & Schuster.

17. Dickinson, E. (2000). Recharge rehab. *Journal of Emergency Medical Services 25* (11), 25–26, 28, 30, 32, 34–35.

18. Cadigan, R. T., & Johnson, S. (1989). *Management guidelines for volunteer ambulance services: a handbook and workbook for managers.* Boston: New England Council for Emergency Medical Services.

19. Donaldson, V. & Donaldson, C. (1998). EMS hero commits suicide. *Journal of Emergency Medical Services, 24* (3), 94–95, 97–100, 103, 105.

FURTHER INFORMATION

Internet Resources

Fun place for personality tests: http://www.tellmemytype.com/

The Web's Stress Management and Emotional Wellness Page: http://www.imt.net/~randolfi/StressPage.html

National Center for PTSD//National Center for Post-Traumatic Stress Disorder: http://www.ncptsd.org/

Interesting perspective on stress: http://stress.jrn.columbia.edu/

A Medical Basis of Stress, Depression, Anxiety, Sleep Problems, and Drug Use:
http://www.teachhealth.com/

Media Resources

Movies
Bringing Out the Dead

Hospital

Mother, Jugs, and Speed

Paramedics

The Doctor

Books
Benson, H., & Stuart, E. M. (1993). *The wellness book.* New York: Fireside.

Canfield, J., & Hansen, M. V. Any of the *Chicken soup for the soul* series.

Covey, S. (1990). *The 7 habits of highly effective people.* New York: Simon and Schuster.

Goleman, D. (1997). *Emotional intelligence.* New York: Bantam Books.

Gray, J. (1992). *Men are from Mars; women from Venus.* New York: HarperCollins.

Heshmat, S. (2001). *An overview of managerial economics in the health care system.* Clifton Park, NY: Delmar Learning.

LaRoche, L. (2002). *Life is not a stress rehearsal.* New York: Broadway Books.

CHAPTER 17

EMS Wellness

Things You Can Do to Help Yourself Handle Stress Better

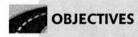 **OBJECTIVES**

Upon completion of this chapter, you should be able to:

- Demonstrate a number of methods you can develop to handle stress.
- Identify certain attitudes that help you better cope with stress.
- Understand that your relationships with other people can help you deal with stress.
- Appreciate the role of exercise and diet both in your wellness and in the way you handle stress.

THE CHALLENGE

Stress is a significant part of the EMS world.[1] As outlined in Chapter 16, there are many sources of stress in the lives of EMS providers. These include the work itself, the hours, the shifts, the time away from families, the schedule, and the daily uncertainties. EMS providers frequently encounter the three D's of stress: *diversion* from an emergency department (ED) because that hospital is full, *depression*—the patients, the situation, and their families are often depressed— and *death* of patients or colleagues. Then there are the indelible, haunting images of horror from scenes such as Oklahoma City and the attack on the World Trade Center, the Pentagon, and a field in Pennsylvania. Pressures are real and do not go away. Yet, there are things one can do to make oneself actually stress resistant.[2] In this chapter we offer a number of specific ways you can prepare for those stresses so that you can deal with them better.

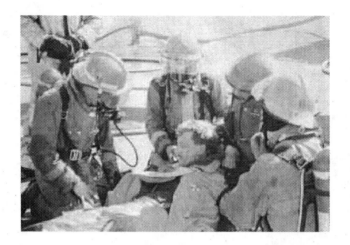

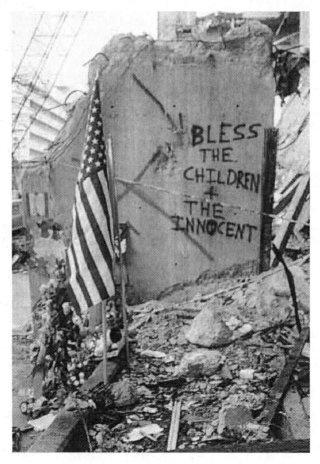

THE EMS PROVIDER AND THE SITUATION

It is the end of the shift and Paul Robinson and Billy Johnson feel it. They have worked hard. They had two minor automobile accidents, a cardiac arrest in the ambulance, and one interrupted almost-sudden infant death syndrome (SIDS) on their run. And, oh yes, they had tons of paperwork to do. They are tired and ready for the shift to end. Both are veteran EMS providers. Both are married with two children each. They appear so similar that other crew members call them "the twins."

Paul heads out the door so quickly he does not even take time to say good-bye. His first stop is at The Purple Cow, his neighborhood's watering hole, where he downs two beers before going home. This stop precipitates harsh words from his wife and annoyance from his children. At supper he takes an extra dessert and is quietly disturbed that he feels like a stranger at a strange table. He sadly notes his weight gain. Then he watches television and retires late to restless sleep. He feels that his lifestyle is wrong but also senses that he is both trapped in his body and life.

Billy departs only after joking with the crew coming on and notes, "Some days the pigeons win; some days, the statues win. Today the pigeons did real well." He also stops to ask Pedro Williams how his son is. Pedro's son has been home for several days with a bad cold. Then, Billy also stops on the way home but his stop is at the gym where he pumps iron for 45 minutes and showers before heading home.

On arrival at his house his wife greets him with a kiss and then the two prepare supper together. Billy's two children acknowledge his entrance with a "hi" and then go back to their activities. As they eat, there is an animated discussion and some good-natured "ribbing about the ribs." Later that night, after Billy helps the kids with homework, he and his wife work on an upcoming church fundraiser. Then they go to bed together. Box 17–1 lists some of the possible results of too much stress on the job.

BOX 17–1

SCOPE

Depression, suicide, substance abuse, and divorce happen all too frequently within the EMS family. To some degree the job stresses contribute to these results.

THE EMS PROVIDER'S WORLD

Paul and Billy face similar daily stresses. Each day they participate in a cavalcade of human dramas and traumas. They see a baby born and watch a man die. They work together and share the everyday trials and tribulations. They are both affected by their job and its experiences. Yet, each handles stress quite differently.

This chapter not only focuses on one's attitude and lifestyle but it also goes one step further. We argue that one's way of thinking and behavior can help a person better deal with these job and life stresses. So we outline a number of ideas and activities that may make a person stress resistant. If you pay attention to your attitude, your feelings, your situation, and your behavior, you can handle the turbulent seas of your life better. (These aspects are summarized in Box 17–2.)

Attitude—Your Way of Thinking

There is a great saying—*your attitude determines your altitude*. It means that how you see your life and the world will influence how you feel and do. For example, if you get up in the morning and see a bleak, terrible day ahead of you, chances are that is the type of day you will have. However, if you are optimistic and upbeat, then you will encounter a good day. In other words, your attitude creates a self-fulfilling prophecy.

The point is that mental posture is one of the key ingredients in how you handle stress. There are two ways of thinking that have been particularly effective and productive in stress management: an attitude of taking command and a stance of being committed to a goal.

Take Command. For many EMS providers, EMS is a matter of responding. They spend all their time responding to demands that are unpredictable and crises that are unexpected. True, but how you react to them and how you

---

BOX 17–2

FOUR ASPECTS OF BECOMING STRESS RESISTANT

1. *Attitude*   Your way of thinking

2. *Feelings*   Your emotional experience

3. *Situation*   The social context of your life

4. *Behavior*   Your lifestyle choices

conduct your life gives you numerous opportunities to take charge. In the crisis itself all your training has geared you to take charge of the chaos. The triage system offers command-decision context. Yet, a take charge attitude is more than that. It involves how you spend you free time. Paul feels like he drifts in the bar. Yet, Billy allots a specific time to keep his body in shape at the gym. Paul just watches television; Billy works on a project. Different ways of *commanding* their time.

Commit to a Goal. Having a goal makes many of life's difficult moments bearable. For example, one EMS provider had as her goal to become a paramedic. For her, aiming at that educational objective made all her rent and roommate problems just "small potatoes" in the grand scheme of things. Perhaps, the simple goal of rearing healthy, productive children takes on a greater meaning if you see kids in trauma. Yet, if you plan to take the family to Disney World or to Hawaii as your goal, then fights over the dirty dishes are placed in a different context.

Feelings—Your Emotional Experience

The emotional experience has two aspects—your feelings and humor. We first focus on feelings and then look at the power of a good sense of humor.

EMS providers' feelings possibly represent one of the most difficult topics in this book. EMS stands for rationally delivered emergency medical care. It means providing the best scientific medical intervention. Yet, the very situations and interventions evoke emotional responses. Feelings are part and parcel of the emergency response.

So let us look at the role of emotions in stress and stress management. However, in this exploration one must be mindful of the fine line that separates denying feelings and being too emotional, which represents the EMS provider's dilemma. For many EMS providers the daily trauma seemingly forces them to not be emotional but to be detached and distant. They react to the everyday drama by emotionally withdrawing; thus, ultimately depriving their patients, their families, and themselves of the feeling quality and "human" aspects of the job.

Furthermore, from a mental health point of view, denied feelings can be devastating to the individual. In a way, hidden feelings constitute an emotional abscess that grows, causes pain, and can burst. Therapy often involves allowing the person to get in touch with his or her feelings and to talk about them. Again, the consequences of keeping "it in" can make EMS providers too detached.

Yet, if EMS providers become too emotional, their feelings can jeopardize the care they provide. Too many feelings can cloud one's clinical judgment or even cause the EMS provider to experience unprofessional reactions. An example of a situation in which becoming too emotional can impair one's clinical judgment involved the following experience. EMS providers were attending a

10-year-old boy who had been struck by a truck as he was riding his bike to school. The EMS providers transported him to the ED and worked as part of the team trying to save his life there. After an hour the ED physician pronounced the boy dead, but one of the EMS providers had a great deal of trouble stopping the resuscitation attempt.

An example of a situation in which becoming *emotional* led to unprofessional conduct occurred when an intoxicated, delirious patient caused a fatal automobile accident. As the EMS provider struggled to place him on the ED bed, the patient hit her in the face. She reacted by slapping the patient. She later explained, "I did not think. I felt hurt and angry."

In addition, if EMS providers are too involved they run the danger of taking all their feelings home with them. Their families feel their pain. In the extreme, their emotions cripple them.

Despite these two dangers—too distant and too emotional—we argue that EMS providers must be aware of their feelings. It is critical that they *can cry* and then they must *stop crying*. They must be able to acknowledge their feelings, share their feelings, and respect and honor these emotions. Paul has difficulty with his feelings. Billy is well aware of his own feelings and is willing to share them with others. Yet, he is in command of their emotions.

The EMS providers in the final analysis must not only be aware of their feelings, but must also realize that they have some control over when and where they express them.

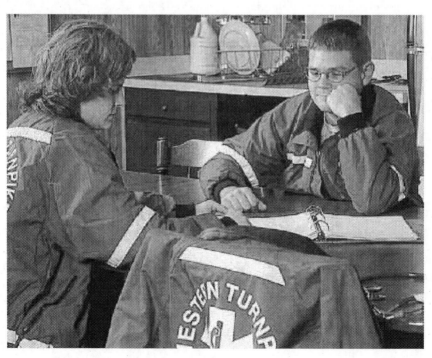

Having a sense of humor represents one of those key ways to handle stress. One of the appeals of the television series *M.A.S.H.* was its use of black humor. In the depth of the combat experience, the crew managed to crack jokes and keep working. Humor also allows you not to take yourself too seriously.

Situation—The Social Context of Your Life

In marked contrast to the first concepts—attitude and feelings—which are self-generated, the social context revolves on the relationship of the person to his immediate and wider community. It involves moving beyond the self. It features your interaction with others. Here, the social context means three key involvements: being with others, seeking others, and concern for others, which are summarized in Box 17–3.

Being with Others. Perhaps, the best way to understand the importance of *being with others* is to look at the history of stress management. The early studies centered on the concept of burnout. Workers became emotionally spent in the job, experienced low morale, and ultimately dropped out. In other words, they were burned out. The literature emphasized that one key condition or symptom leading to staff burnout was *isolation*. Thus, these individuals started to avoid their colleagues. They ate alone. They rarely socialized with others, and they withdrew from nonessential interactions. They might simply have been seen reading quietly over in the corner or just never seemed to be around at all.

The point here is that *not being with others* represents an indication of isolation. Isolation is the key ingredient in burnout. Putting a positive spin on isolation, being around your coworkers, helps to prevent burnout. Furthermore, of historical interest, the concept of stress management replaced burnout because of the negative connotation of that term. Burnout means management has already lost the staff. Stress management suggests there are things management can do with the staff in order to prevent burnout.

Finally, isolation provides an important indicator to EMS providers. Namely, if you observe a colleague starting to withdraw from others, consider that that person is becoming burned out. Your attention to that individual can reverse the isolating process.

BOX 17–3

THREE KEY SOCIAL CONTEXT INVOLVEMENTS

1. Being with others
2. Seeking others
3. Concern for others

Seeking Others. In contrast to being with others, *seeking others* has an action connotation. In this situation the person actively goes out, engages, and meets with other people. It also has the distinct quality of the initiator enjoying the interaction. Again, look at the difference between Paul and Billy. At the end of the shift, Paul avoids others and simply leaves. Billy likes his coworkers

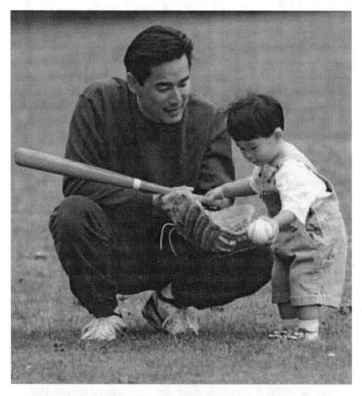

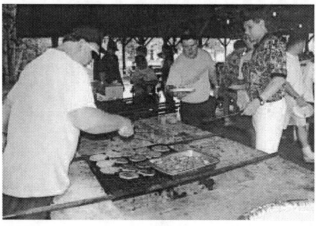

and the other emergency personnel. He seeks out Pedro to inquire about his son. He clearly represents a person who likes others.

Concern for Others. Finally, there remains the basic reason people seek careers in EMS—a *concern for others*. However, that concern must not only be for your patients but it also must extend to others—your coworkers, your family, and your community. Billy is interested in his coworkers, his family, and his community.

Behavior—Your Lifestyle Choices

Up till now we have emphasized steps you can take mentally, emotionally, and socially to become stress resistant. We now focus on a series of lifestyle behaviors that will better prepare your body and *therefore your mind* for stress. Clearly, the mind and body are incredibly intertwined. Activities such as diet and exercise not only strengthen your body but also improve your mental abilities. We concentrate on the two key actions—exercise and diet (Box 17–4).

Together exercise and diet represent actions you can do for and by yourself. One of the earlier ideas—"Take command"—directly applies here. Diet and exercise work directly and beneficially for your body's health but they also allow you to feel in charge of your life. Thus, by choosing a proper diet and exercise you move from the position of victim of stress to a person with some control over his life. Billy feels great both physically and mentally after working out and he has a sense of making a great selection for the use of his time.

After approval by your physician, we recommend that you engage in a 20 to 60 minute aerobic exercise program at least three times or more a week (Box 17–5).[3] Such a program means doing a sustained workout period. Aerobic exercise burns off fats; anaerobic exercise burns carbohydrates. Your program could be tennis, jogging, weight training, cycling, walking, swimming, dancing, squash, racket ball, stair climbing, basketball, or soccer. The benefits of such a regime are legion and legend.[1] These benefits include lowered blood pressure, lowered pulse, increased cardiac muscle strength, better coronary collateral circulation, enhanced cardiorespiratory fitness, stronger bones, better muscle tone and strength, weight loss, increased mental accuracy, increased energy, enhanced sense of well-being and an improved sex life among other things. Finally, the bottom line is that after you are finished exercising you simply feel better.

BOX 17–4

TWO KEYS TO LIFESTYLE CHOICES

1. Exercise
2. Diet

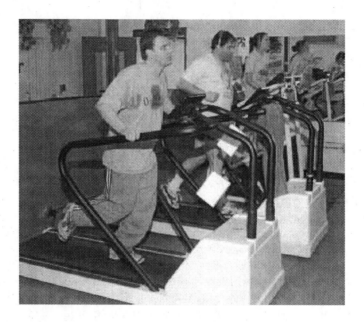

BOX 17–5

EXERCISE

20–60 minutes of aerobic exercise three or more times per week is recommended.

Diet consists of two parts—what you put into your mouth and what you do not put into your mouth. This means consuming less red meats; less fats, especially those that are saturated, less carbohydrates, more minerals and vitamins, and more fruits and vegetables. Your diet should translate into eating less and sharper. Your lifestyle change should also include no nicotine, moderate alcohol use, and no abused substances. As with exercise, you not only eat better but also have a sense of control of your diet.

CONCLUSION

Thus far we have treated attitude, feelings, situation, and behavior as separate. In reality, if you combine them, they are even more effective. For example, if you jog with a partner, you can talk about issues, gain some social interaction, and decrease isolation. Furthermore, by exercising you generate endorphins, which in turn promote an optimistic attitude. Eating with colleagues or your family means social interaction and support as well as checking isolation.

REVIEW QUESTIONS

1. Define attitude and discuss its relationship to handling stress.
2. What are feelings and how do they relate to stress?
3. Review ways that working and talking with your colleagues can help with stress.
4. What is the difference between aerobic and anaerobic exercise?
5. Discuss the role of diet in dealing with stress.

EXERCISES

1. Make a list of methods you and your colleagues have used effectively to handle stress.
2. List your life goals.
3. Take a 1-mile walk with your colleague. Then discuss the effects of that walk on you. You will be amazed at the things exercise can do.
4. Keep a log of your exercise and diet activities for one week. This record will indicate patterns of exercise and food intake.
5. Sit quietly alone for 20 minutes and then review your reactions to this period.

REFERENCES

1. Beebe, R. W. O., & Funk, D. L. (2001). *Fundamentals of emergency care.* Clifton Park, NY, Delmar Learning.
2. Flannery, R. B., Jr. (1990). *Becoming stress resistant through the project SMART program.* New York: Continuum.
3. Hoeger, W., & Hoeger, S. (1999). *Principles and labs for physical fitness* (2nd ed.). Englewood, CO: Morton Publishing Company.

FURTHER INFORMATION

Internet Resources

Alcoholics Anonymous: www.alcoholics-aonymous.org

American Cancer Society: www.cancer.org

American Heart Association: www.amhrt.org

Avoiding weight gain after stopping smoking: www.ash.org

Improving your marriage: www.competentcouples.com

National Institute of Mental Health: www.nimh.nih.gov

Sticking to an exercise program: www.primusweb.com/fitnesspartner

Weight management: www.weight.com

Media Resources

Wellness Movies

My Big Fat Greek Wedding

Chariots of Fire

Any Marx Brothers movie

Save the Last Dance

Patch Adams

Shrek

Books

Cooking and Diet

Peeke, P. (2001). *Fight fat after forty*. New York: Penguin.

Weight Watchers' new complete cookbook. New York: Pearson Education Macmillan.

Fitness Books

Connelly, A. S. (2001). *Body rx*. New York: G. P. Putnam's Sons.

Kara, J. (2001). *The business plan for the body*. New York: Three Rivers.

Laliberte, R., George, S. C., & Men's Health Editors. (1997). *The men's health guide to peak conditioning*. Emmaus, PA: Rodale Press.

Payne, W. A., & Hahn, D. B. (2000). *Understanding your health* (6th ed.). Boston: McGraw-Hill

Uplifting, Insightful, and Motivational Books

Benson, H. (1975). *The relaxation response*. New York: Avon Books.

Canfield, J., & Hansen, M. V. *Chicken soup for the soul* series. Deerfield Beach, FL: Health Communications.

Carlson, R. (1997). *Don't sweat the small stuff and it's all small stuff*. New York: Hyperion.

Fulghum, R. (1986). *All I really need to know I learned in kindergarten*. New York: Ivy Books.

Harris, T. A. (1969). *I'm OK—you're OK*. New York: Avon Books.

Morgenstein, J. (1998). *Organizing from the inside out.* New York: Owl Books.

Redfield, J. (1997). *The Celestine prophecy.* New York: Warner Books.

Rose, R. (2000). *The complete idiot's guide to living together.* Indianapolis, IN: Alpha Books.

Answers to Review Questions

Chapter One

1. Emotions and thoughts generally precede and explain observed behavior.
2. Patients may behave in ways that EMS providers find baffling. It is important to approach the scene without preconceptions.
3. Observe, Interact, Ask, Act, Attend, Document.

Chapter Two

1. Among the controllable factors are: high-fat diet, smoking, obesity, high blood pressure, diabetes.
2. Denial, fears such as loss of job, delay in seeking help.
3. They may feel guilty for creating anxiety or for not having done more before the symptoms occurred.
4. The open-ended question allows for a more detailed assessment of the patient's level of consciousness and organization of thought.
5. Onset, Provocation, Quality, Region, Radiation, Relief, Severity, Timing. This acronym can be used to gather assessment data on all patients.
6. Negative reactions can include developing a protective delusion of invincibility, retreating to technical care, freezing, or developing sarcastic humor.

Chapter Three

1. The growing elderly population presents with a vast array of physical and emotional problems.
2. Senescence is the process of growing old. There are significant changes in all of the body's systems and in many activities of daily living.

3. Depression, memory loss, and fatigue.

4. Ageism is acting on the basis of stereotypes rather than responding to the older patient as a person. It can show up in interaction and in value judgments that a careless EMS provider might let slip into documentation.

Chapter Four

1. Denial, anger, bargaining, depression, acceptance.

2. It may create tension among family members at a time when the patient most needs support.

3. Fear of death or fear of spreading disease may lead some EMS providers to attempt to distance themselves from the possibility by joking about it.

4. Following standard precautions is appropriate in all patient care situations.

5. Seek to understand the person who is speaking. Listen to tone and inflection as well as choice of words. Pay attention to body language. Don't rush to judgment. Make it clear that you have understood the person when you respond.

Chapter Five

1. A patient may feel mortified by having his or her clothes cut away. A patient may envision the loss of important self-defining activities—even independence. A patient may fear a disfiguring injury.

2. If one party sees the other as responsible, it can affect the future relationship.

3. Abstraction, pity, "professional warmth," compulsive hyperactivity.

4. Documenting multiple sets of vital signs, trauma scores, and mental status exams will help hospital staff evaluate changes in the patient. Lack of establishing a trend or details of the mechanism of injury could impact on the care the patient receives once at the hospital.

Chapter Six

1. The victim may feel a greater sense of vulnerability or distrust of others.

2. It may be difficult to talk about the experience to the police. Repeating the story may cause the victim to relive the assault. The rapist might be an acquaintance or even a spouse. The victim might be an undocumented resident.

3. Reactions include: powerlessness, numbness, disbelief, embarrassment, shame, guilt, depression, and disorientation.

4. A medical examination is necessary to determine if the victim has been physically injured. It is necessary to ease fears about disease, pregnancy,

and so forth. It is essential to collect evidence in case the victim decides to prosecute.

5. The victim has been robbed of autonomy by the assault. Bringing the victim into the decision-making process can help to reinforce her autonomy.

Chapter Seven

1. Stress and alcohol or other drug abuse.

2. Victims of parental aggression may inflict aggression on their own children.

3. The child may be chronically sad and emotionally blunted. The child may feel responsible for the abuse.

4. Persons with ideas of reference; persons who are easily overwhelmed; perfectionists; persons who were themselves abused as children.

5. The parents may not be cooperative. Young children may not have a good understanding of cause and effect.

6. Focus on the child's need for medical care. Do not attempt to be a social worker or family therapist.

7. Good documentation can make the case for follow-up treatment.

Chapter Eight

1. Gradual buildup of emotion; free-floating anxiety; delusions and hallucinations; self-medication; social settings that encourage violent behavior.

2. Don't handle a violent patient on your own. Use all your senses in approaching the situation. Slow down. Convey an image of quiet reassurance. Don't take angry statements personally. Label emotions appropriately. Maintain appropriate eye contact. Pay attention to nonverbal cues. Never ask "Why?" questions. Reinforce positive behavior.

3. Retreat from the scene and immediately call for police assistance.

4. Retreat from the scene and call for police assistance to secure the weapons and the scene.

Chapter Nine

1. Normal activities of daily living such as altered sleep patterns, eating disorders, hypersexuality, use of alcohol and other drugs are disrupted. These changes can have a dramatic effect on health.

2. A depressed person may feel that it is necessary to hurt others.

3. A depressed patient can exhaust a family.

4. Yes. It can help you assess the level of risk.

5. Never leave the patient alone. Secure the patient appropriately during transport. Make sure that the patient does not have access to potential weapons.

Chapter Ten

1. Alcoholics deny, minimize, and rationalize their behavior.
2. Codependents can provide support or excuses for the alcoholic's drinking. A codependent family member may reduce the patient's motivation for treatment.
3. Alcohol-related accidents; intentional traumas; alcohol-related illnesses; withdrawal-related conditions; pathological intoxication; inebriation itself.
4. Clearly identify yourself; do not use derogatory or overly familiar nicknames; make it clear that you are not law enforcement; emphasize physical concerns.

Chapter Eleven

1. Drug and alcohol use; social rejection; mental illness.
2. Chronic mental illness, hypothermia; skin conditions; liver disease.
3. Drug intoxication; inadequate personality may affect communication, but do not assume the patient cannot participate in treatment.

Chapter Twelve

1. The patient may attempt to banter with the EMS provider.
2. The patient may insist on detailed explanations of everything the EMS provider does.
3. The patient may focus on symptoms during the examination and may tend to cling to helpers.
4. The seductive patient may seek attention to gratify needs (unlike many patients who are in need of help). The litigious patient may seek support for his or her allegations. The somatizing patient may present as weaker or sicker.

Chapter Thirteen

1. The United States has become more ethnically and religiously diverse. This trend is expected to continue into the future.
2. Stereotyping is seeing all members of a particular group as the same. Prejudice is seeing people who are different from oneself as being inferior. Discrimination is acting on the basis of prejudiced and ethnocentric attitudes.

3. EMS providers must recognize their own feelings but act professionally.

4. Be aware of ethnic and religious differences and similarities. Use translators if necessary. Ask questions respectfully. Be aware of discomfort in the patient's reactions. Document carefully, without stereotyping.

Chapter Fourteen

1. Denial and isolation, anger, bargaining, depression, and acceptance.

2. The family may be unprepared for loss. Grief can be overwhelming. Responses can include grief, anger, depression, self-deprecation, and physical pain.

3. Among other situations, EMS providers may need outside support when they feel they may be responsible in some way; when they know the deceased; and when the victim is a child.

Chapter Fifteen

1. Warning, threat, impact, inventory, rescue, remedy, and recovery.

2. Panic and paralysis are two common behavioral responses. Emotionally, these physical reactions are associated with emotional release and emotional shutdown.

3. Fear of being overwhelmed. Concern for their own families.

4. Planning is essential. EMS providers should know their roles in advance. It is important that everyone knows what to expect from other public safety agencies at the scene.

5. Stress-related physical responses; problems in relationships.

Chapter Sixteen

1. The responses are opposites: withdrawal or overinvolvement.

2. The EMS provider may experience a sense of persistent sadness, chronic anxiety, indifference or distance, or an emotional high from emergency activity.

3. No. Stress may promote personal growth and change.

4. Emergency medical work is psychologically demanding. Shift work places stress on families.

5. To answer this question, you must first do an appraisal of your lifestyle. Are you an active person or do you prefer more reflective activities such as reading? Then, apply your style as a management technique. For example, active folks often find exercise like jogging or swimming as very effective ways to handle stress. If you like more quiet methods then you might find meditation, or attending movies, or yoga as your stress management vehicle.

Chapter Seventeen

1. Attitude is one's mental posture. Two aspects of attitude are especially important: being in control of the situation and being committed to a goal.

2. Feelings are emotional reactions. The EMS provider who denies feelings and the EMS provider who does not channel them appropriately can each impair his or her ability to provide care and to manage stress effectively.

3. Being with others in social activity reduces the tendency to burnout. Seeking others out will build moral–social capital. Concern for others has a positive effect on one's own sense of self.

4. Aerobic exercise burns fat; anaerobic exercise burns carbohydrates. Aerobic exercise lowers blood pressure, lowers pulse, increases cardiac strength, aids in weight loss, increases mental accuracy, increases energy, gives one an enhanced sense of well-being, and improves sex life.

5. Increasing intake of minerals and vitamins and fruits and vegetables, and decreasing alcohol, and eliminating nicotine and illicit drugs improves stress-handling capacity.

Glossary

Acquired immunodeficiency syndrome (AIDS): the final stage of infection with the HIV virus.

Acute myocardial infarction (AMI): the death of heart muscle due to an inadequate supply of oxygen-rich blood.

Affect: the emotional reactions to a situation; the conscious, subjective part of an emotion, as opposed to the body's physical reaction.

Ageism: prejudice and discrimination against a person based solely on that person's elderly status. For example, not hiring a person because he or she is over 65 years old.

Alcoholism: dependence on drinking alcoholic beverages; characterized by long-term excessive use of alcoholic beverages and impaired social and vocational functioning.

Ambivalence: uncertainty; holding two contradictory attitudes toward a person or idea at the same time.

Angina: pain or discomfort that is the result of insufficient oxygenated blood flow to the heart muscle.

Anxiety: fear or uneasiness about an anticipated event; in psychiatric terminology, anxiety is fear or apprehension not connected to a specific event and accompanied by such physiological signs as sweating, increased heart rate, and hypertension. To stress the lack of connection between the emotion and any known cause, the condition is sometimes referred to as free-floating anxiety.

Aura: the subjective sensations, such as flashes of light, a distinctive smell or taste, or even an emotion, that signal the onset of a seizure or migraine. See also **prodromal.**

Autonomy: independence; self-government; the state of being able to make one's own choices.

Cadence: a rhythm to the measure of voice.

Cauliflower ear: deformity of the ear due to tissue damage and regrowth of repaired tissue.

Codependence: the state of condoning and in some ways sharing a family member's or loved one's dependence on alcohol, drugs, or addictive, self-destructive behavior. The codependent husband of an alcoholic may not drink, for instance, but his own emotional needs and psychological problems lead him to continue the relationship and thus encourage the behavior.

Congestive heart failure (CHF): a condition in which there is a backup of pressure from the left ventricle, allowing fluid to leak out of the pulmonary capillaries and into the alveoli.

Coronary heart disease (CHD): any disease process that impedes flow of oxygen to the heart, weakening the heart muscle.

Coup-contrecoup: French for "blow-counter-blow"; trauma to an area caused by the rebound of tissue from a blow to another area. For instance, in an automobile collision, the passenger's head strikes the windshield; the initial trauma is to the brain's frontal lobe, and the coup-contrecoup injury occurs when the occipital lobe rebounds against the posterior skull.

Cynicism: distrusting the actions and motives of others; a belief that people generally act out of selfishness.

Defensive medicine: overanalyzing or overtreating a patient because of the fear of a lawsuit.

Delirium: mental confusion often associated with disorientation, hallucinations, and aimless activity.

Delirium tremens: a delirium caused by withdrawal from alcohol in an alcohol-dependent person. Sometimes referred to as "the DTs," delirium tremens may occur 3 to 5 days after the patient has stopped drinking. Marked by fever, disorientation, hallucinations, and sometimes seizures, delirium tremens is a serious medical condition with a significantly high risk of mortality.

Delusion: a false belief held by a person in spite of physical evidence to the contrary and opposed to the person's own experience and information.

Dementia: a loss of mental ability due to the loss of neurons or brain cells.

Depression: an emotional state marked by feelings of sadness, hopelessness, and worthlessness; the onset of depression is accompanied by alterations in sleep habits, appetite, work, and sexual activity.

Discrimination: acting on one's prejudices. People have feelings about others. In discrimination one actually acts on these feelings. For example, one may dislike gays. That is prejudice. Not renting an apartment or hiring a person because he or she is gay is discrimination. Discrimination is illegal.

Distraught: experiencing emotional distress, doubt, and conflicting thoughts. Feeling distraught is common to people faced with sudden, severe loss, such as the death of a loved one.

Do not resuscitate (DNR) order: legal document that specifies the actions that can be taken by health-care providers in the event of a life-threatening emergency.

Dysphoria: clinical term for unhappiness, particularly sudden, unexplained depression, restlessness, and dissatisfaction.

Ego ideal: a view of one's self based on what one would like to be or what one considers a hero or ideal to be.

Elder at risk: an elderly person who has a mental condition, for example, dementia, or a physical problem, such as inability to ambulate, which puts that individual at risk for injury. That problem warrants further assessment and possibly intervention. Most states have programs to respond to elders at risk and some states provide adult protective workers to help those elders.

Erythropoietin: hormone that triggers red blood cell production.

Ethnocentricity: seeing one's own group—religious, ethnic, geographic, or sexual—as being superior to others.

Euphemisms: use of flowery language and expressions that are unclear and beat around the point.

Flat affect: an apparent lack of emotional responsiveness, characterized by monotone voice and lifeless eyes. See also **affect.**

Free-floating anxiety: See **anxiety.**

Grandiosity: an unrealistic, inflated sense of self-importance, wealth, power, or status.

Hallucination: an untrue perception that has no basis in reality and is not based on actual stimuli; a person can hallucinate by seeing, feeling, hearing, or tasting something that is not there.

Hallucinosis: a condition in which the person is experiencing hallucinations but remains oriented and with intact intellect. In alcoholic hallucinosis, the person is withdrawing from alcohol and having hallucinations, usually of an auditory type, with clear intellectual functions.

Hepatitis B   an infectious disease caused by the Hepatitis B virus that can result in permanent damage to the liver.

Human immunodeficiency virus (HIV):   a virus that causes malfunction of the immune system, rendering the victim unable to adequately ward off viruses; it is the viral agent that causes AIDS.

Hyperactivity: a childhood disorder marked by excessive, constant activity; difficulty in learning and concentration; and, sometimes, disruptive behavior.

Hyperreflexia: a condition of excessively sensitive and exaggerated reflexes; a symptom of increased nervous system reactivity.

Hypersomnia: getting an excessive amount of sleep.

Hypochondriac: an individual who is obsessive about his or her health; excessively worrying about symptoms and ailments.

Ideas of reference: a person's delusional suspicion or belief that certain events—a television program, an overheard conversation, the flight of a bird—have special meaning directed only to him or her. For instance, a woman who believes that Dan Rather, reporting on homelessness, is telling her to give away all her belongings, is suffering from ideas of reference.

Illusion: a mistaken perception or misinterpretation of sense impressions, differing from hallucination in that it is based on actual stimuli. When the illusion is fixed—that is, when the person cannot or will not correct the misinterpretation when it is pointed out—it is a delusion. See also **delusion.**

Impulsivity: the tendency to act on impulse, without forethought or planning.

Incident command system (ICS): a management system used on the emergency scene that is designed to maintain order and follow a sequence of set guidelines.

Insomnia: inability to get an adequate amount of sleep.

Korsakoff's psychosis: a personality disorder that frequently occurs with chronic alcoholism and is characterized by disorientation, delirium, insomnia, hallucinations, and pain in the extremities.

Labile: this describes an emotional content that often changes dramatically—for example, from sad to very happy, and then to apathy, and then happiness again. These fluctuations are frequently unrelated to events.

Learned helplessness: feeling and acting helpless in all situations as an ingrained response due to always being treated as though one is helpless.

Litigious: inclined to engage in lawsuits.

Lucid: having a complete sense of self and surroundings; able to make clear speech.

Mandated reporters: individuals who come into contact with certain situations, for example, child abuse, and are required by law to report these situations to the proper authorities.

Melting pot: term used to describe the makeup of American society since people from various countries all immigrated and chose to live in America as one unified group.

Multiple casualty incident (MCI): an event in which patient needs exceed EMS system resources.

Paradoxical: contrary to expectations. A *paradoxical reaction* to medication is opposite to the desired reaction; for instance, some patients become aggressive after administration of a mild tranquilizer.

Paranoia: a psychiatric disorder marked by persistent, systematic delusions of persecution; also, in general terms, unwarranted suspicion or jealousy.

Pathological intoxication: a condition in which there is an excessive reaction to moderate doses of alcohol, possibly including violent behavior and amnesia concerning the episode.

Post-traumatic stress: inability to cope with an extremely stressful situation that occurred in the past but that is continuing to provoke anxiety and fear in present activities, adversely impacting on one's daily life.

Preconceptions: preformed beliefs about an individual, a place, or a situation; prejudice or bias.

Prejudice: seeing others and other groups that are different from oneself as not only different but also as inferior.

Presbycusis: diminished hearing acuity with age.

Presbyopia: diminished visual acuity with age.

Prodromal: before the outbreak of disease; referring to the period between the earliest indications of a disease and the appearance of the major symptoms. *Prodromal symptoms,* like the aura some people experience before seizure, signal the onset of illness. See **aura.**

Psychosis: extreme mental disorder marked by the disintegration of personality and loss of contact with reality.

Regression: responding to stress (e.g., physical illness or psychiatric disorder) by resuming behaviors, emotions, or thought patterns from an earlier stage of personal development.

Schizophrenia: a major, chronic, mental disorder; a psychosis marked by disruptions in and disconnections between thoughts, emotions, and behaviors. Symptoms may be positive (delusions, hallucinations) or negative (ambivalence, regression, withdrawal).

Self-medicating: using medications to treat one's perceived illnesses or problems without a physician's prescription.

Senescence: the natural process of aging. It does not imply pathology. For example, graying hair with age is senescence.

Seroconversion: the response of the immune system's antibodies to a vaccine or disease-causing agent.

Sexually provocative: tending to arouse sexual interest in others through dress, language, gesture, or other behaviors.

SIDS: sudden infant death syndrome.

Somatizing: expressing a mental condition (neurosis, anger, personality conflict) as a bodily disorder.

Stereotype: the view of seeing all people of a certain group, all Latinos or Jews or Asians, in a certain way. For example, in this stereotype, one sees all Arabs as terrorists.

Syncope: a passing loss of consciousness.

Thought block: the abrupt termination of a thought process, as when an individual suddenly stops his or her line of reasoning and does not resume it; this behavior is frequently seen in schizophrenia.

Tossed salad: new term used to describe the makeup of the United States as a country of people with a variety of backgrounds, beliefs, religions, and customs.

Vignette: a fictional short story.

Index

Abused child, 75–88
  challenges, 75–79
  patient and situation, 76–79
    behavior of patient, 80–81
    considerations for EMS
      providers, 86
    emotions and thoughts behind
      behavior, 81–82
    family/bystander responses,
      81–82
    intervention strategies, 84–86
    patient's world, 79
    provider responses, 83–84
Abuser, 79
  personality types, 81
Acting, 7
Active listening, 170
Activity disruptions accompanying
    depression, 109–110
Acute myocardial infarction, 11
Addicts, 124
Ageism, 27
AIDS (acquired immunodeficiency
    syndrome), 39–49

  challenges, 39–40
  patient and situation, 40–42
    behavior of patient, 43
    considerations for EMS
      providers, 86
    emotions and thoughts behind
      behavior, 43–44
    family/bystander responses, 44
    intervention strategies, 45–47
    patient's world, 42
    provider responses, 44–45
AIDS-related complex (ARC), 42
Alcohol, 124
Alcohol abuse, 119–132
  challenge, 119–120
  patient and situation, 120–122
    behavior of patient, 123–124
    considerations for EMS
      providers, 129–130
    emotions and thoughts behind
      behavior, 124–126
    family/bystander responses,
      126
    intervention strategies, 127–129

Alcohol abuse (*cont.*)
  patient's world, 123
  provider responses, 126–127
Alcoholics, 123
Alcoholics Anonymous, 126, 130
Alcoholism, 2
Anger, 93
Angina, 15
Anxiety, 3, 16, 93–94
Armed patient, 100
Asking, 7
Attending, 7
Attitude, 220–221
Autonomy, 71, 79

Becknell, John, 8
Beebe, R., 100
Behavior of patient, 4
Being with others, 223
Black out, 125
Bray, G., 201
Bystander responses, 5

Cadence, 33, 34
Cardiac emergency, 11–22
  challenges, 11–12
  patient and situation, 12–14
    behavior of patient, 15
    considerations for EMS
      providers, 20
    emotions and thoughts behind
      behavior, 16
    family/bystander responses,
      16–17
    intervention strategies, 17–20
    patient's world, 14–15
    provider responses, 17
Cardiopulmonary resuscitation
  (CPR), 17

Cauliflower ear, 85
Challenges facing EMS, 1–2
Child abuse. *See* Abused child
Child victim, 79
Churchill, Winston, 160
Codependents, 123, 126
Coles, Robert, 2
Communication
  face-to-face, 170–171
  family, 211
  with patient, 3–4
Concern for others, 225
Congestive heart failure, 11
Considerations for EMS providers, 8
Coronary heart disease (CHD), 11
Coup-contrecoup injury, 58
Covey, Stephen R., 47, 209
Critical incident stress debriefing
  (CISD), 59, 184, 197, 208,
  211–212
Cynicism, 3

Death in ambulance, 177–188
  challenge, 177
  patient and situation, 178–180
    behavior of patient, 181–182
    considerations for EMS
      providers, 186
    emotions and thoughts behind
      behavior, 182
    family/bystander responses,
      182–183
    intervention strategies,
      184–186
    patient's world, 181
    provider responses, 183–184
Defensive medicines, 154
Delirium, 31, 44
Delirium tremens, 99

Delusion, 94, 124
 of invincibility, 20
Dementia, 31, 44
Denial, 16
Depression, 2, 31
Depression and suicide, 105–117
 challenge, 105–106
 patient and situation, 106–108
  behavior of patient, 109–110
  considerations for EMS
   providers, 115
  emotions and thoughts behind
   behavior, 110–111
  family/bystander responses,
   111–112
  intervention strategies, 113–115
  patient's world, 109
  provider responses, 112–113
Designer drugs, 130
Diet, 225–226
Discrimination, 164
Distraught person, 75
Diversity, 163, 173
 paradox, 169
Documenting, 7
Dodson, D., 197
Do not resuscitate (DNR) order,
 184, 186
Drugs, 130
Dysphoria, 110

Education, 209–210
Elder at risk, 33
Elderly, 23–38
 challenges, 23–24
 patient and situation, 25
  behavior of patient, 27, 30
  considerations for EMS
   providers, 35–36

emotions and thoughts behind
 behavior, 30–31
family/bystander responses,
 31–32
intervention strategies, 32–35
patient's world, 26–27
provider responses, 32
population statistics, 23–24
Emotions behind behavior, 4–5
Employee assistance programs
 (EAPs), 130, 208
Employee assistance referrals, 212
EMS providers, considerations for, 8
Enabler, 79
Epidemiologic studies, 59
Erikson, Erik, 79
Ethnocentricity, 164
Euphemisms, 33
Exercising, 225

Face-to-face communication,
 170–171
Family communication, 211
Family responses, 5
Fatigue, 31
Feelings, 221–223
Fisher, R., 208
Flashbacks, 205
Flat affect, 137
Free-floating anxiety, 16
Funk, D., 100

Getting to Yes (Fisher and Ury), 208
Gloving, 45
Goal, 221
Grandiosity, 94

Hallucinate, 44
Hallucinations, 94, 124, 125

Hallucinosis, 99
Head trauma, 56
Health maintenance, 209
Hepatitis B, 40, 44, 45
HIV (human immunodeficiency
    virus) infection, 39
Homeless people, 133–142
    challenge, 133–134
    patient and situation, 134–136
        behavior of patient, 137
        considerations for EMS
            providers, 141
        emotions and thoughts behind
            behavior, 137–138
        family/bystander responses, 138
        intervention strategies,
            139–140
        patient's world, 136
        provider responses, 138
Humor, 20, 223
Hyperactivity, 79
Hyperreflexia, 124
Hypersomnia, 31
Hypochondriac, 7, 143, 156, 157

Ideas of reference, 80
Illusion, 124
Impulsivity, 55
Incident command system (ICS),
    191
Inebriate, 123
Insomnia, 31
Interacting, 6–7
Interpersonal space, 171
Intervention strategies, 5–7
    act, 7
    ask, 7
    attend, 7
    document, 7

interact, 6–7
observe, 6
Isolation, 223

Journal, 210–211

Korsakoff's psychosis, 127
Kübler-Ross, E., 43, 181

Labile blood pressure, 25
Learned helplessness, 167
Life interests, 209
Lifestyle choices, 225–226
Listening effectively, 46
Litigious patient, 148–154
    patient and situation, 148–151
        behavior of patient, 151
        bystander responses, 152
        considerations for EMS
            providers, 159
        emotions and thoughts behind
            behavior, 152
        intervention strategies, 153
        patient's world, 151
        provider responses, 151
Lucidity, 32

Management practices, 210
Mandated reporters, 75
Manic individuals, 94
May, Rollo, 81
Medical history, 19, 99–100
Melting pot, 167
Memory loss, 31
Mental illness, and homelessness,
    137
Mission statement, 209
Multiple casualty incident (MCI),
    189–199

challenge, 189–190
patients and situation, 190–192
  behavior of patients, 194
  considerations for EMS
    providers, 197–198
  emotions and thoughts behind
    behavior, 194–195
  family/bystander responses, 195
  intervention strategies, 196–197
  patients' worlds, 192
  provider responses, 195

Observing, 6
OPQRST method, 18, 20
Overinvolvement, 203

Paradoxical behavior, 93
Paranoid patient, 152
Paranoid reaction, 98
Pathological intoxication, 127
Patient, potentially violent. *See*
    Potentially violent patient
Patient and situation scenarios, 2–3
  behavior of patient, 3–4
  considerations for EMS providers,
    8
  emotions and thoughts behind
    behavior, 4–5
  family/bystander responses, 5
  intervention strategies, 5–7
  patient's world, 3–4
  provider responses, 5
Patient's world, 3–4
Persons in pain, responding to, 60
Pets, 35
Post-traumatic stress, 8
Potentially violent patient, 89–103
  challenge, 89
  patient and situation, 90–93

behavior of patient, 93
considerations for EMS
  providers, 101–102
emotions and thoughts behind
  behavior, 93–95
family/bystander responses,
  95–96
intervention strategies, 96–101
patient's world, 93
provider responses, 96
Preconceptions, 5
Prejudice, 164
Prodromal period, 93
Provider responses, 5
Provocative patients, 143–161
  challenge, 143–144
  litigious patient, 148–154
  seductive patient, 144–148
  somatizing patient, 154–159
Psychotherapy, 212

Rape, 63–74
  challenges, 63–64
  patient and situation, 64–66
    behavior of patient, 67
    considerations for EMS
      providers, 72–73
    emotions and thoughts behind
      behavior, 68–69
    family/bystander responses,
      69–70
    intervention strategies, 70–72
    patient's world, 67
    provider responses, 70

Regression, 147
Relationships
  with other professionals, 211
  among workers, 211

Responding to all people, 163–175
  challenge, 163–165
  patient and situation, 165–166
    behavior of patient, 167
    considerations for EMS
      providers, 173
    emotions and thoughts behind
      behavior, 167–168
    family/bystander responses, 168
      encouraging assistance, 168
      passively blocking care, 168
      preventing help, 168
    intervention strategies, 169–172
    patient's world, 166–167
    provider responses, 168–169
Rockwell, Norman, 169

Schedules, 211
Schizophrenic patient, 94
Seductive patient, 144–148
  patient and situation, 144–146
    behavior of patient, 146
    bystander responses, 147
    considerations for EMS
      providers, 159
    emotions and thoughts behind
      behavior, 146–147
    intervention strategies, 148
    patient's world, 146
    provider responses, 147–148
Seeking others, 224–225
Self-destructive acts, 110
Self-medication, 94
Self-protection, 101
Senescence, 27, 28–29
Seroconversion, 39
Seven Habits of Highly Effective People,
    The (Covey), 47, 209
Sexually provocative patient, 4

Social context, 223–225
Somatizing patient, 7, 154–159
  patient and situation, 154–156
    behavior of patient, 157
    bystander responses, 158
    considerations for EMS
      providers, 159
    emotions and thoughts behind
      behavior, 157–158
    intervention strategies,
      158–159
    patient's world, 156–157
    provider responses, 158
Stereotyping, 46, 164
Stress, 201–215
  Challenge, 201–215
  situation, 202–203
    emotions and thoughts behind
      behavior, 204–206
    EMS providers' behavior, 203
    EMS provider's world, 203
    family/workplace responses,
      206–207
    intervention strategies,
      207–208
      intervention, 208
      recognition, 207–208
      timing, 208
    specific intervention methods,
      209–212
    early intervention, 210
    individual early-intervention
      strategies, 210–211
    later-intervention strategies,
      211–212
    management early-
      intervention strategies,
      211–212
    prevention, 209–210

Substance-abusing patient, 123
Suicide. *See* Depression and suicide
Super-EMS provider, 203
Syncope, 25
Syrus, Publius, 128

Thought blocking, 138
Thoughts behind behavior, 4–5
Torrey, E. Fuller, 134
Tossed salad concept of diversity,
    168
Translator, 170
Trauma, 51–62
   challenges, 51–52
   patient and situation, 52–54
      behavior of patient, 55
      considerations for EMS
         providers, 59–60
      emotions and thoughts behind
         behavior, 55–56
      family/bystander responses,
         57
      intervention strategies, 58–59

patient's world, 54–55
provider responses, 57–58
Triage, 194

Unwanted people. *See* Homeless
    people
Ury, S., 208

Vignette, 2
Violence. *See* Potentially violent
    patient

Waeckerle, Dr. Joseph, 195
"War of the Worlds" broadcast, 194
Wellness, EMS, 217–229
   challenge, 217
   EMS provider and situation, 219
   EMS provider's world, 220
      attitude, 220–221
      behavior, 225–226
      feelings, 221–223
      social context, 223–225
Withdrawal, 203